THE SENSORY PROCESSING DISORDER

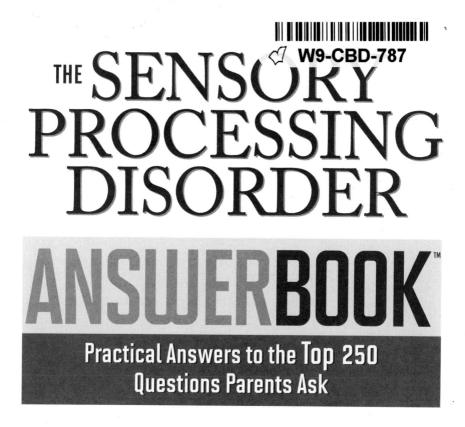

ANSWERBOOK™

Practical Answers to the Top 250
Questions Parents Ask

TARA DELANEY, MS, OTR/L

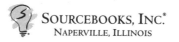

SOURCEBOOKS, INC.®
NAPERVILLE, ILLINOIS

This publication is designed to provide accurate and authoritative information in regard to the subject matter covered. It is sold with the understanding that the publisher is not engaged in rendering legal, accounting, or other professional service. If legal advice or other expert assistance is required, the services of a competent professional person should be sought.—*From a Declaration of Principles Jointly Adopted by a Committee of the American Bar Association and a Committee of Publishers and Associations*

This book is not intended as a substitute for medical advice from a qualified physician. The intent of this book is to provide accurate general information in regard to the subject matter covered. If medical advice or other expert help is needed, the services of an appropriate medical professional should be sought.

All brand names and product names used in this book are trademarks, registered trademarks, or trade names of their respective holders. Sourcebooks, Inc., is not associated with any product or vendor in this book.

Published by Sourcebooks, Inc.
P.O. Box 4410, Naperville, Illinois 60567–4410
(630) 961–3900
Fax: (630) 961–2168
www.sourcebooks.com

Library of Congress Cataloging-in-Publication Data

Delaney, Tara.
   The sensory processing disorder answer book : practical answers to the top 250 questions parents ask / By Tara Delaney.
      p. cm.
   Includes bibliographical references and index.
   1. Sensory integration dysfunction in children. 2. Sensory integration dysfunction. I. Title.
   RJ496.S44D45 2008
   618.92'8—dc22
                              2008012929

Printed and bound in the United States of America.
BG 10 9 8 7 6 5 4 3

Contents

Acknowledgments

I owe a deep thanks to June Clark of Fine Print Literary Agency for her dedication to her writers and her openness to ideas, as well as her intellectual insight. Your spirit and passion for life are infectious!

Thanks to Sara Appino, my editor at Sourcebooks, for offering valuable advice and truly "welcoming" all the answers on Sensory Processing Disorder.

To all my colleagues and friends in the therapy and research world who I learn from every day, I am in constant awe of your skill, commitment and ability to inspire and help kids. To the faculties at the University of Texas Health Science Center and the University of Wisconsin Occupational Therapy schools: I owe a debt of gratitude to you for equipping me with knowledge as well as inspiring me to seek answers.

To the team at BabySteps, your professionalism and commitment to children touch me. Thanks to Mary Hamrick, Director of Speech Therapy, for all the brainstorming sessions and your desire to make life better for the kids we serve.

Thanks to the Donaghy, Delaney, McPhillips and McCaghey clans for encouraging creativity and seeing possibilities.

I am truly grateful to my three sisters, Heather, Megan, and Megan, for thinking I can do anything! To my parents, Julie and Denis McCaghey, thanks for your unceasing love. Mom, you believe everything I write is important, and of course the world will want to read it! Dad, you taught me that failure only comes when you quit, so keep going.

Thanks to Maggie and Liam, my children, for teaching me that questions and answers are lived and learned. My greatest gratitude goes to my husband Bill for making my passion his and devoting many late hours to reading and reworking ideas. You are a gift.

Introduction

It's interesting how life is... I have been a pediatric occupational therapist for fifteen years. I specialize in Sensory Processing Disorder, as well as autism spectrum disorders, in my private practice, BabySteps, a pediatric therapy and educational services company. Because I teach sensory processing courses to fellow therapists, educators, and parents, I am asked a broad range of questions that I record and incorporate into my practice and courses. As life would have it, those questions and answers are more pertinent to my life than I could have imagined.

In 2004 I adopted a little girl from China. All those questions I was asked as an occupational therapist were now mine as a parent, because I now had a child with sensory "issues." Questions such as: Why doesn't she like to be cuddled? We're supposed to bond! Why does she arch away from me—doesn't she like me? Why does she scream when she gets near water? Babies are supposed to love water! How can I parent a child who is afraid of everyday sensations?

Even as the questions flooded my brain, the answers, *my answers,* were sitting right there. Seeing my child struggle with everyday sensory information drove me to organize the wide body of knowledge floating around about Sensory Processing Disorder into a coherent and useful answer book.

This book systematically endeavors to answer some of the most common, as well as unusual, questions about Sensory Processing Disorder and how it impacts our children's lives. I attempt to answer all the pertinent questions about what sensory processing is, how to tell when it is not functioning properly (Sensory Processing Disorder), and what you, as a parent, can do about it.

Chapter 1

WHAT IS SENSORY PROCESSING DISORDER?

- What is sensory processing?
- What is Sensory Processing Disorder?
- What causes SPD?
- What are some of the general signs of Sensory Processing Disorder?
- Who "discovered" SPD?
- What percentage of the population has Sensory Processing Disorder?
- I've heard it called *Sensory Integration Dysfunction* and *Sensory Processing Disorder*. Which is it?
- What are the three categories of Sensory Processing Disorder?
- What is Sensory Over-Responsivity?
- What is Sensory Under-Responsivity?
- What does *sensory seeking* or *craving* mean?
- What are the Sensory Based Motor Disorders?
- What is Postural Disorder?
- What is Dyspraxia?
- Don't we all have some sensory "issues"?
- Is Sensory Processing Disorder a real diagnosis?
- Can a child have SPD without having another diagnosis?
- Can a child have SPD in addition to another diagnosis?
- Do more boys suffer from sensory processing difficulties than girls?
- It seems like Sensory Processing Disorder is on the rise. Is that true?
- Can you see sensory processing difficulties in an infant?
- How early can you detect sensory defensiveness processing disorder and treat it?
- Is there a cure for SPD?
- Are all sensory processing disorders the same?
- I was told to take my son to an occupational therapist. What is that?

Q. What is sensory processing?

A. *Sensory processing* or *sensory integration* refers to the nervous system's job of taking in all the information around us through our senses (movement, touch, smell, taste, visual, and hearing) and organizing that information so that we can attach meaning to it and act on it accordingly. Sensory integration is the basis for learning. It is what allows us to get an idea of what is going on in the world around us. We learn when we take in new information, cross reference the new information to previous similar experiences, and make an assessment as to how we should proceed given the current set of information.

For example, when you hear a dog barking, your ears take in the information and your brain attaches meaning to it, such as identifying it as an animal, not a cat but a dog, determining how close it is, and deciding whether it sounds like a big dog or a small dog. Then the brain matches that information with past experiences that have been stored as memory. If you have ever been bitten by a dog, you may run to get away when you hear the barking. On the other hand, if you grew up with dogs, the sound may make you homesick for your childhood home.

The development of sensory systems begins in the womb and continues throughout our lives. In the early childhood years, the nervous system is in hyper-development and sensory integration is being refined through typical childhood activities. This is why the first few years of childhood are considered the sensory-motor years, and are crucial for laying the foundation for our nervous system.

Q. What is Sensory Processing Disorder?

A. Sensory Processing Disorder (SPD) describes the difficulty that some people's nervous systems have in making use of and integrating sensory information. SPD can exist when there are no other underlying conditions or can be present in conjunction with other neurological or psychological diagnoses.

Q. What causes SPD?

A. Sensory Processing Disorder is a result of neurological disorganization that affects nervous system processing in a few different ways. The brain is not receiving messages, or the messages that are received are inconsistent, or the sensory information is consistent but does not integrate properly with other sensory information from the other related sensory systems.

Q. What are some of the general signs of Sensory Processing Disorder?

A. Here is a list of signs that may point to Sensory Processing Disorder:

- Overly sensitive to touch, movement, sights, or sounds
- Underreactive to touch, movement, sights, or sounds
- Easily distracted
- Social and/or emotional problems
- Activity level that is unusually high or unusually low
- Physical clumsiness or apparent carelessness
- Impulsive, lacking in self-control
- Difficulty making transitions from one situation to another
- Inability to unwind or calm self
- Poor physical self-concept
- Delays in speech, language, or motor skills
- Delays in academic achievement

Q. Who "discovered" SPD?

A. Sensory Processing Disorder (originally called *Sensory Integration Dysfunction*) was first "discovered" in the mid-1900s but was not given any attention until Dr. Jean Ayres, an occupational therapist, psychologist, and neuroscientist, wrote a book called *Sensory Integration and Learning Disabilities* in 1972. The book was based upon research that linked sensory processing to learning difficulties. Building upon Dr. Ayres's work, other researchers and therapists drew a link between sensory processing difficulties and behavior.

Q. What percentage of the population has Sensory Processing Disorder?

A. A recent study showed that at least 5 percent and up to 13 percent of the population has Sensory Processing Disorder.

Q. I've heard it called *Sensory Integration Dysfunction* and *Sensory Processing Disorder.* Which is it?

A. Beginning in the 1970s, the term *Sensory Integration Dysfunction* was commonly used. However, as the field matures and we learn more about how sensory processing difficulties can manifest themselves differently in children, there has been a need for a more expansive term that has evolved into the term *Sensory Processing Disorder.* You will still hear the term *Sensory Integration Dysfunction* occasionally.

The term *sensory integration* is mostly reserved for explaining how the nervous system *processes* sensory information, whereas *Sensory Processing Disorder* describes the condition that reflects *difficulties with how we register and process* that information. Sensory Processing Disorder is an umbrella term covering three categories, which will be discussed extensively in the next question.

Q. What are the three categories of Sensory Processing Disorder?

A. 1. Sensory Modulation Disorder (SMD)

Sometimes the nervous system's reactions to everyday stimuli are either "too much" or "too little" relative to the stimuli. Sensory

Modulation Disorder describes this set of conditions. There are three subtypes of SMD:

- Sensory Over-Responsivity Disorder
- Sensory Under-Responsivity Disorder
- Sensory Seeking/Craving

2. Sensory Discrimination Disorder (SDD)

One of the key things the sensory nervous system does is give us vital information about our own bodies as well as our environment. Sensory Discrimination Disorder is the inability to distinguish one type of input from another. Persons with SDD have difficulty distinguishing and categorizing various attributes about the physical environment. A child may not process hot and cold in the same way we do or may not process the difference when lifting a full soda can versus an empty one.

3. Sensory-Based Motor Disorders

These disorders result when a child's nervous system is not processing or integrating movement and body information, leading to interference with a child's motor skills. Sensory Based Motor Disorders have two subtypes:

- Postural Disorder
- Dyspraxia

Q. What is Sensory Over-Responsivity?

A. Sensory Over-Responsivity (SOR) describes a condition of the nervous system characterized by outsized responses to stimuli. SOR is probably the type most people associate with SPD. You will probably hear therapists and others refer to Sensory Over-Responsivity as *sensory defensiveness*.

SOR is an aversive reaction to sensory stimuli that others perceive as pleasurable or that stay below the "irritation radar." Usually SOR is associated with the sense of touch. For example, most of us do not register the touch sensation from the seams of our socks or the tags on our shirts. Our bodies' "touch" system has habituated to these sensations so they do not distract us as we go about our day. People who are sensory defensive to touch are so distracted by these sensations that they can be consumed by them and be unable to concentrate on anything else until the sensation is removed. That is why you hear stories about the tags being cut from the clothing of children who are sensory defensive.

Q. What is Sensory Under-Responsivity?

A. Sensory Under-Responsivity (SUR) describes a condition of the nervous system characterized by less than typical sensory response to stimuli. As a result, the child does not appear to process and respond to sensory information such as noise, movement, or touch. For example, you may see this child putting a loud toy against his ear because he requires increased amounts of auditory and/or vestibular input, or he may be flapping his hands in front of his face in order to get some visual information, or he may appear completely unaware of his own body and hug others too hard. These children are often sensory seekers because they are not registering typical amounts of input the way you or I do, so they seek a greater quantity and intensity of sensory information in order to register it and process it.

Q. What does *sensory seeking* or *craving* mean?

A. Sensory seeking/craving is when a person's nervous system requires unusual or intense amounts of stimulation. This is the kind of kid who crashes into things, or takes a lemon and sucks on it, or who may even bite himself, or is constantly touching things to get more input. This child "just can't get enough" sensory information.

Q. What are the Sensory Based Motor Disorders?

A. Sensory Based Motor Disorders result when a child's nervous system is not processing or integrating movement and body information so that it interferes with a child's motor skills. Usually these children appear uncoordinated or clumsy. The sensory processing disorders are broken down into two separate categories, Postural Disorder and Dyspraxia—described in the next two questions.

Q. What is Postural Disorder?

A. Postural disorder is characterized by children who have difficulties maintaining appropriate body postures for any given motor task, moving, and sedentary activities. This is a child who exhibits low muscle tone and will get tired easily. For example, a child with postural disorder would get tired even while trying to maintain upright posture at a desk. This is different than motor planning difficulty (dyspraxia), which is the lack of ability to plan how to do an activity. A child with postural disorder may be able to plan how to do an activity but will not be able to maintain postural control to actually carry out the activity.

Q. What is Dyspraxia?

A. In children with dyspraxia, there is a breakdown in one or more of the steps required for motor skills, which impacts a wide range of activities. "Praxis" is the complicated set of steps your brain and body take to get something done. Praxis relies on our sensory systems working effectively. Difficulties with praxis usually reflect underlying sensory processing problems. Praxis is not something you either use or don't use; we utilize praxis more when we are performing a novel activity and less when it is something we have done millions of times. Most of the time we are unaware of or only slightly aware of this process. It takes the following steps:

1. **Ideation:** Simply, this is knowing what to do and having some idea of how to go about doing it. This is part of the function in play when you set out to perform or even think about performing a sequence of complex movements, especially new ones—for instance, learning a new dance.

2. **Planning:** This is the process your brain and body go through to determine how to do something—for instance, how to move your feet for the new dance. This process is active throughout an activity since the brain and body are constantly revising the planning phase in order to accommodate new information, such as what your partner's feet are doing or the beat of the music. Often, when people use the term *motor planning*, they are referring to the whole process of praxis. Motor planning is the second step of praxis.

3. **Execution:** This is the body's ability to act on the idea and the planning that went on in the brain. Execution is dependent upon an extensive amount of communication between the brain's motor centers (motor cortex) and the muscles—for example, moving your feet and hands gracefully to all the new dance maneuvers.

Children with dyspraxia may have the following characteristics:

- Difficulties with fine motor skills for arts and crafts, scissor activities, and handwriting

- Difficulties with gross motor skills, such at throwing, kicking, or catching a ball, or jumping with both feet off the ground
- Difficulties with activities that require bilateral coordination (the use of both hands together for one activity)
- Always reluctant or refuses to try a new activity
- Insists on being last for familiar or new motor activities
- Acts like the class clown who is always falling or tripping
- Has difficulty imitating movements for games such as "Simon says"
- Does not follow verbal directions for motor movements well
- Often lacks ideas for play

Q. Don't we all have some sensory "issues"?

A. The simple answer is yes. Many of us experience sensory processing difficulties. How much we are affected is often dependent on what is going on in our lives. For example, when you are under extreme stress and you are not sleeping well, you may use artificial ways to keep yourself alert, such as caffeine, and you may feel yourself becoming overly sensitive to noise or touch. Sensations that seemed pleasurable last week (your son singing the ABCs) are now annoying to your ears, so much so that you want to yell, "PLEEEEASE, no more ABCs!" Since you understand the sensation is temporary and you don't want to hinder your son's expression, you simply clench your jaw.

Many women can relate to increased sensory-nervous system sensitivity during their monthly cycle. Hormones affect the neuro-chemicals that directly act on a woman's nervous system, which can make women less able to modulate normal, everyday stimulation during this time of the month. Many women will have reactions to seemingly ordinary experiences, such as touch, smells, or noise, that shouldn't make them feel like crawling under a table, but they can't help how their bodies feel. Those of you who have been pregnant have probably experienced sensory overload a number of times during your pregnancy (smells, anyone?).

The most important thing to remember is that what you experience is usually temporary or can be altered through changes in lifestyle, such as using less caffeine and getting more exercise. However, for those who have SPD, controlling these reactions is difficult, bordering on almost impossible.

Q. Is Sensory Processing Disorder a real diagnosis?

A. Yes and no. Sensory Processing Disorder is not yet part of the *Diagnostic and Statistical Manual* (DSM) used by the American Psychological Association, which does list other diagnoses, such as autism, depression, and bipolar disorder. It can take years for a condition to make it into this manual. For example, Asperger's syndrome was not entered into the DSM until 1994, although it was first identified in the 1940s by Hans Asperger. There is a movement currently under way by the Sensory Processing Network and other groups to have SPD entered into the DSM.

Sensory Processing Disorder has been recognized by parents and therapists for more than thirty years. Sometimes the diagnosis is a secondary diagnosis. For example, a child may have autism as the primary diagnosis with a secondary diagnosis of Sensory Processing Disorder. (FYI: The medical community refers to a secondary diagnosis as a *co-morbid* diagnosis.)

It is important to be aware that because SPD is not part of the DSM yet, medical professionals seeking a diagnosis will often misdiagnose a child with SPD as having attention deficit-hyperactivity disorder (ADHD), depression, anxiety, or something else that is considered an "official" diagnosis. This is one of the reasons the occupational therapy community feels so strongly about having SPD included in the DSM. The hope is to prevent children who have sensory processing difficulties from being misdiagnosed and help them get the right treatment.

Q. Can a child have SPD without having another diagnosis?

A. Since sensory processing disorder is considered a neurological impairment, there is always a chance that there could be other neurological underpinnings that are in part responsible for the sensory processing difficulties. Some of the more common traceable causes of SPD are mild brain damage during birth, premature birth, lack of sensory exposure (such as occurs with institutionalized children), and environmental factors such as fetal alcohol exposure. It could also be linked to a diagnosis of Fragile X, autism spectrum disorder, attention deficit disorder (ADD), and ADHD.

Q. Can a child have SPD in addition to another diagnosis?

A. Yes. Because SPD is not yet an official diagnosis, medical professionals often do not think to consider SPD as a possible answer to difficulties a child is having. There is a strong chance that SPD will be overlooked and another diagnosis will be given. Also, a child could have a primary diagnosis of autism or ADHD and have a secondary diagnosis of SPD.

Note: Children may be misdiagnosed with ADHD or ADD or other diagnoses when the underlying reasons for the behavior stem from difficulties with sensory processing. This is discussed in further detail in Chapter 14.

Q. Do more boys suffer from sensory processing difficulties than girls?

A. As with most of the neurologically based diagnoses (autism, Asperger's syndrome, and ADHD), boys do not fare as well as girls, and sensory processing disorder is no different. My experience and the reports of many of my colleagues show that boys are referred to occupational therapists much more often than girls. Although boys do seem to be more affected than girls, "boy behavior" may be mistaken for a sensory difficulty, and some behaviors commonly attributed to girls may mask a sensory issue. For instance, boys tend to seek out more intense sensory stimulation, so a boy's normal behavior may be perceived, incorrectly, as SPD. On the other hand, a girl who is less coordinated or has lack of control of her body may pull back or sit on the sidelines but will tend to be viewed as simply not interested in physical activities, although the reason she does not participate is due to SPD.

Another reason that boys are perceived as having sensory processing difficulties is the fact that most boys do not develop fine motor skills or visual motor skills as early as girls. As a result, they often struggle with fine motor and visual motor demands, such as writing, copying information from a board, using a scissors, and all the other activities we use to judge our children's academic abilities in the early grades. These difficulties may result in a boy being referred to occupational therapy in the schools.

Q. It seems like Sensory Processing Disorder is on the rise. Is that true?

A. In the last few years, I have seen a large increase in the number of referrals related to sensory processing disorder. Several of my colleagues report the same pattern. There may be several reasons for this. First, society as a whole is becoming more aware of sensory processing and how certain behaviors may be explained by a child's difficulty with processing sensory information.

Second, our lifestyles are changing. Over the last twenty years, we have become an "indoor" society, so that most of our work and, more important, most of our entertainment, is located indoors. This means our children's brains and bodies are not as involved in the activities that promote healthy nervous system development. Many therapists and others in the medical field believe that changes in lifestyle are contributing to the rise in difficulties our children are experiencing. The good thing about this is that we can combat some of these effects by incorporating activities that promote healthy nervous system development into our children's lives.

Q. Can you see sensory processing difficulties in an infant?

A. Yes, but parents may not understand that certain behaviors they see in their infant can actually be SPD. Often it is not until the child is older and a therapist starts asking questions about that child's behavior as an infant that the picture becomes clear.

Here are a few tell-tale behaviors that may suggest an infant is having difficulties processing sensory information:

- Is unable to be consoled by others
- Arches away when someone holds him
- Screams when being rocked
- Prefers to be laid in the bed and calm himself to sleep instead of being rocked and cuddled
- Has difficulties with sucking and breastfeeding
- Does not exhibit normal pain reactions, such as crying when given a shot
- Has an aversion to water or certain textured clothes that other infants find soothing

Infants with SPD are more prone to having trouble settling into a normal sleep/wake cycle. Parents also report other behaviors, such as an infant who constantly bangs his head against the bed or sits and rocks incessantly.

Motor activities may also be hindered in an infant with SPD. An example is a child who should be reaching and grabbing things but keeps his hands fisted and close to his sides. These infants might not use both hands together to hold a bottle, crawl, or pull themselves to standing within the developmental range for this skill.

If you suspect that something is not quite right with your child's development, a pediatric therapist should examine your infant to determine if it is SPD.

Q. How early can you detect sensory processing disorder and treat it?

A. Since there is no blood test, chromosomal test, or any other concrete medical test that can detect SPD, the way we determine if someone has SPD is by documenting a portfolio of behaviors, then grouping those behaviors to point to a diagnosis of SPD.

When we look at an infant, we want to make sure to rule out any kind of medical concern that may be contributing to certain behaviors and then look toward the infant's nervous system development and make determinations. This may involve time and certain determinations. If you have questions about your infant's development, it will not hurt to contact a therapist and find out ways to help your child. You may be offered very simple ideas to try with your infant that will help your child and you!

Q. Is there a cure for SPD?

A."Cure" is a strong word. Research is fairly young in this field, so we have no longitudinal studies that would tell us if a child with SPD is actually cured. Longitudinal studies are designed so that researchers can follow a group of people for many years to look at the long-term impacts of a certain procedure, disease, or treatment. We do know from anecdotal studies and documentation that children with SPD who receive intense therapy and learn self-coping mechanisms are more successful academically and socially. Also, science tells us that nervous system development continues into adulthood and our experiences certainly impact that development. It is reasonable to assume that providing a nervous system with experiences that aid in healthy integration is going to have long-term benefits. It is important to note that when an occupational therapist works with a child with sensory processing disorder, the therapist is not simply treating the sensory issues but rather targeting that child's "occupational deficits" that are impacting his or her life.

Q. Are all sensory processing disorders the same?

A. No. Like most other things, Sensory Processing Disorder is different in each person. Effective processing of sensory information is dependent on all seven senses working properly and being able to work in conjunction with each other. Thus, there are many ways that Sensory Processing Disorder may be seen in sensory-nervous system processing. Furthermore, each child will react differently to neurological processing difficulties.

Q. I was told to take my son to an occupational therapist. What is that?

A. Occupational therapists can be thought of as the professionals trained to be the ambassadors between your nervous system's processing of information and your actual functional abilities. Their goal is to help their patients lead independent, productive, and satisfying lives. They work with individuals who have conditions that are mentally, physically, developmentally, or emotionally disabling. They help these individuals develop, recover, or maintain daily living, play and work/academic skills. Occupational therapists help clients improve their basic motor functions and reasoning abilities and compensate for permanent loss of function.

Chapter 2

UNDERSTANDING SENSORY INTEGRATION

- What happens in the body during sensory integration?
- Can you give an example of how sensory integration works?
- Does sensory integration happen differently for each person?
- Are there really more than five senses?
- What exactly are the seven senses?
- How do the sensory systems work together?
- What is the vestibular sense?
- How do you know when the vestibular system is working?
- How does the vestibular sense develop?
- What are the common signs of vestibular difficulties?
- Is the tactile sense more than touch?
- How does the tactile system develop?
- What are the common signs of tactile difficulties?
- What is the proprioceptive sense?
- How can I experience the proprioceptive sense?
- What are the common signs of proprioceptive difficulties?
- What is the visual sense?
- What are visual skills?
- How does the auditory system work?
- What are the common signs of auditory processing difficulties?
- What is the gustatory system and how does it work?
- What is the olfactory sense and how does it work?
- What are common signs of olfactory/gustatory difficulties?

Q. What happens in the body during sensory integration?

A. Your body is equipped with sensory receptors located throughout your body, such as those in your ears and eyes as well as in joints and tendons. These sensors are designed to take in the information from your environment, as well as information about what your body is doing at any given time. The information gathered by your sensory receptors travels as electrical impulses by way of millions of neurons that create a path to areas in the brain designed to interpret that information. The brain decodes and categorizes the information by matching it with past stored information and attaching meaning to it. The sensory systems work together to create a whole picture of your environment. The brain sends a message via neuro-pathways back to the areas in the body (and other parts of the brain) that react to incoming stimuli.

Q. Can you give an example of how sensory integration works?

A. You are walking in the forest and take in the deep, crisp smell of pine after a morning rain. Your nose (the sensor) takes in the information (the smell molecules). The information is converted to electrical impulses that travel through your olfactory nerve (a nerve that registers smells). The information is delivered to the part of the brain responsible for decoding the information, called the olfactory bulb. The brain then conducts a matching game to past smells.

Your smell sensory system actually shares more direct neural connections with the memory and emotion center of your brain (called the hippocampus) than any other sense. That is why smells often have such a powerful emotional connection. For me, the smell of pine takes me back to being a little girl in Wisconsin and going camping with my dad on Lake Tahoe. This is a positive memory for me, so my output is a flood of positive neurochemicals in the brain, resulting in an overall content and happy feeling.

Q. Does sensory integration happen differently for each person?

A. The process works the same for everybody, but the interpretation of the information is different for each person. When everything is working properly, the information travels in the same way in each person to the same centers of the brain. The difference is in the way the brain melds new information with past stored information to give it context. This difference results in our individual perception of a given experience or stimuli.

Let's say that many years ago, you dated a guy who wore Brut cologne (which also has a deep pine scent, as in the previous example). The guy turned out to be a jerk and the relationship ended badly. So when you take in that deep scent of pine, your brain likely conjures up that jerk of an ex-boyfriend, and the result is an uncomfortable feeling that makes you want to wince. This is a very different reaction from the positive feelings brought on by the same scent in the previous example.

Q. Are there really more than five senses?

A. Yes. In school, we are taught that there are only five senses: smelling, hearing, seeing, touching, and tasting. This is logical, because we are highly aware of these five senses (technically referred to as the extero-senses) and can easily relate to where they come from and how they are used in our everyday lives. But there are also two hidden senses (intero-senses) that are just as crucial to our daily lives: the proprioceptive sense (body position sense) and vestibular sense (balance motion sense). These senses give us useful information about our body position, the speed of our movement, or objects in our environment, as well as a sense of where we are in relation to everything around us. The proprioceptive sense and vestibular sense work with the touch sense to lay the foundation for the development of the other senses. These foundation senses work together, behind the scenes, to give us an overall feeling of well-being in the world, as well as in our own skin. We become acutely aware of these senses when they are not working, because it knocks us for a loop and makes everyday life challenging.

Q. What exactly are the seven senses?

A. The following table describes each of the seven senses.

Name of Sense	Type of Sensation
Vestibular (body motion)	Bearings in space; balance; where we are relative to the ground and other objects. It is our three-dimensional "you are here" marker, and is the most powerful sensory system.
Proprioceptive (body position)	Body awareness; tells us where our body parts are relative to other body parts and how they are moving relative to each other; the "left hand knows what your right hand is doing" sense
Tactile	Touching sense; gives us information about things contacting the body; tell us about pressure, temperature, texture, size, shape, movement, pain
Visual	Seeing sense; gives us information about the location, color, shape, and distance of objects from one another as well as movement of objects/people
Auditory	Hearing sense; allows us to locate, capture, and discriminate sounds
Olfactory	Smelling sense; one out of two "chemical" senses; gives us information about the odors around us by sensing the chemicals floating in the air
Gustatory	Tasting sense; the second of our "chemical" senses; gives us information about the things that enter the mouth by detecting certain chemicals.

Some therapists also include internal processing, such as digestion, as an eighth sense.

Q. How do the sensory systems work together?

A. The brain is a wonderfully complex organ that is able to take input from all of these systems simultaneously and put them together to give us a complete picture of our environment. The brain requires input from all the sensory systems to create a workable map of what is going on around us and to formulate a desired response.

Let's say you are trying to hit a baseball. Your ears are going to hear the cheering and coaching, your eyes are intent on the ball coming at you, and your vestibular, proprioceptive, and tactile systems are coordinating your body (using the input from your eyes tracking the ball) to time your swing and hit the ball. When you hit a home run, you can thank your nervous system for allowing you to be a hero.

Q. What is the vestibular sense?

A. The vestibular sense is our most powerful and most crucial sense. It may be easier to think of it as the "balance and movement" sense. It answers the question, "Where am I in relation to the earth's surface?" The vestibular sense lets you know whether you are upright, horizontal, moving, or falling by receiving stimuli from the force of gravity through receptors in the inner ear. This information is then sent to your brain for processing. Your brain sends the information about where your body is in relation to the ground directly to the nerves that communicate with the muscles responsible for keeping your body upright.

The balance and motion system receives stimuli from semicircular canals in the inner ear that are sensitive to both the direction of gravity and to motion. These sensors are oriented 90 degrees from each other, which is what allows them to give information about three dimensions. When these receptors are activated, the information is sent to your brain for processing.

Q. How do you know when the vestibular system is working?

A. This question is best answered by the fact that you certainly know when it's *not* working. Have you ever had an ear infection that caused you to be off balance when you stood? That is an unsettling feeling because little else matters when you are unable to stand.

You know the vestibular system is working because of your instant and unconscious understanding of where your body is in relation to the things around it. For instance, when you tilt your head to the side, how do you know your body is still upright? How do you know your feet are still touching the earth when you walk? This sense tells us whether we are standing still or moving, or if objects around us are motionless or moving. It also tells us if we're going forward or backward, walking or running.

If you want to become more aware of this sense, here's an age-old trick. Spin around as fast as you can, then suddenly stop. The tiny currents keep going for a little bit, giving you the sensation that you are still spinning, but in the opposite direction. Your brain compensates for this and causes you to fall, or, at the very least, feel dizzy. You have just become "aware" of your most dominant sense!

Q. How does the vestibular sense develop?

A. The vestibular sense begins developing in utero and continues to develop throughout childhood. A newborn baby already demonstrates responses to gravity and movement. If you hold a baby in your arms and then suddenly lower her, her arms and legs will extend out quickly. This is because the canals in her inner ears are telling her she is falling and she'd better do something quickly. Her brain alerts her muscular-skeletal system, and her arms and legs respond by quickly extending. This reaction is the beginning of what will mature into a protective extension response needed in order to become safely upright and mobile.

The vestibular system develops through the natural progression of childhood movements, which allows it to become increasingly refined in its relationship to gravity. Since development of the vestibular system has relied on our drive to move and explore our environment, children who aren't able to move, or who seldom move because of environmental reason, may not have a well-integrated vestibular system.

Q. What are the common signs of vestibular difficulties?

A. Underdeveloped vestibular systems can impact higher-level skills, as well as coordination, sense of direction, eye control, attention, and aspects of language development. Several academic skills rely on a healthy vestibular development.

Here are some common challenges you may see in a child with vestibular processing difficulties:

- Avoids playground equipment that involves movement
- Avoids activities that require balance
- Fearful of ascending/descending stairs
- When an infant, arches backward when held or moved
- Clumsy, trips easily
- Avoids feet leaving the ground/uncomfortable in elevators
- Poor sense of rhythm
- Becomes overly nauseated from motion

Q. Is the tactile sense more than touch?

A. Yes. The tactile sense is the largest sense we have, with receptors covering the body on the skin. It is a multifunctioning sense that we all need in order to learn about ourselves and the environment around us. Touch tells us about the physical properties around us. It is through touch that infants and children learn the early fine motor skills that are paramount to a sound academic beginning. For example, a child learns that a square has four flat sides, that water is wet, and that she has to grasp a crayon with just the right amount of pressure so it does not break as she makes marks on a piece of paper. She has to be able to feel an object, judge the density of an object, and know how to manipulate it well before she is able to know how to hold a pencil and form the letters of the alphabet.

The tactile sense is broken into two systems. The first system, which is crucial for survival, is the protective/defensive system. This system alerts us to potentially harmful touch, usually light touch, such as from a spider. This is the main sense at work when a child is first born, evidenced by how easily newborns "startle." The second system is the discriminative system. Within a few months of birth, the discriminative system steps ahead as the dominant touch sense. It tells us if, when, where, and how we are being touched. This is the system we rely on when we are touching something to give us information about the physical properties of an object, such as whether it's smooth or rough, hot or cold.

Q. How does the tactile system develop?

A. Starting in utero, the nervous system and the brain work together to create an extensive library of touch experiences. The brain and body are amazingly efficient at storing the memory of those touch sensations. The brain deciphers and catalogues the information, allowing us to make assumptions about other objects or animals with similar properties.

Q. What are the common signs of tactile difficulties?

A. If the touch sense is not developed properly, a child can display difficulties at school with skills such as coloring, cutting, and drawing. A child may also demonstrate behavior problems since he may respond to touch in a negative way or refuse to touch many of the materials related to art projects. He may need to touch every-thing and anything he can, which is often viewed by teachers as impulsiveness, or an ability to follow directions.

Here are some other common challenges you may see a child with tactile processing difficulties:

- Avoids certain textures and materials (clothing, art projects, etc.)
- Is over/underresponsive to normal touching
- Touches everything in sight (sometimes by licking)
- Avoids standing close to others in a crowd (or stands too close)
- Clothes always have to fit "just right" (no seams out of place, etc.)
- Reacts negatively to unforeseen touch
- Cannot identify objects through touch
- Likes to be in tight spaces (wrapped in blanket)
- A picky eater

Q. What is the proprioceptive sense?

A. The proprioceptive sense gives us information about how we are moving and where our limbs are in relation to our own bodies. The main purpose of the proprioceptive sense is to provide body position awareness and to aid in motor control and motor planning.

Proprioceptive receptors are in the muscles, joints, ligaments and tendons, and connective tissue. These receptors are continuously sending messages to the brain about our body's position even when we are not moving.

While reading this, you are most likely seated, legs crossed or out in front, sitting forward or leaning back in the chair. Whatever your body's position, your muscles, joints, and tendons are firing messages to your brain, letting it know what's going on with your body. You don't have to think about your position at any given moment, unless you are performing a new motor skill.

Q. How can I experience the proprioceptive sense?

A. Here is a way to get a feel for how the proprioceptive system works: Shut your eyes and move your hand away from your body. Then move it behind your back, lay it on your knee, and touch your head. Did you ever think about how your body was able to move your hand without your eyes guiding it? Your proprioceptive system was hard at work, giving your brain information about your body without relying on the eyes. We are able to move without conscious thought, which lets us do self-care tasks, such as dressing ourselves, without thinking about every move our limbs are making.

Q. What are the common signs of proprioceptive difficulties?

A. When our proprioceptive system is not working properly, everyday activities such as dressing, sitting up in a chair, or shaking someone's hand with the appropriate amount of pressure can take a tremendous amount of thinking. This can make everyday activities exhausting and onerous.

Here are some common challenges you may see in a child with proprioceptive processing difficulties:

- Has difficulty maintaining postures, even while sitting in a chair
- May appear confused as to how to move her body
- Has a wide stance when standing still
- Uses too little/too much pressure when hugging
- Sits in the "W" position (knees bent in front with legs out to side, giving a wide base of support)
- Falls or crashes into things purposefully
- Grinds teeth/bites or chews objects
- Preferred motion is short and quick, instead of sustained-endurance activities

Q. What is the visual sense?

A. The visual sense encompasses more than just our eyes. While our eyes allow us to see, they are simply the sensory receptors that respond to optical information. Optical information causes the eyes to create an impulse that is transmitted by way of the ocular nerve to the various parts of the brain that decode, decipher, and store the information. This allows the brain to give us a "picture" of what the world looks like. The end part of that process is your brain and body deciding how to respond to the information, whether by lifting your hand to catch a ball moving quickly toward you, responding to the colors on a canvas that create an image that you find pleasing, or physically responding to the dimensions of the rocks as you walk across a brook.

As evidence that we "see" with more than just our eyes, it is quite possible for someone to be completely blind yet have perfectly functioning eyes. In such cases, lack of sight is due to damage or malfunction of parts of the brain responsible for processing visual information. On a similar note, a child can have perfect vision but still struggle with skills that require visual processing, as well as visual skills such as reading, tracking a ball, and navigating one's self in a busy mall.

Q. What are visual skills?

A. Many visual skills beyond visual acuity (the ability to see clearly) lay the foundation for a child's academic and social success.

Binocular vision, or eye teaming, is foundational to the visual system. Difficulties with binocular vision impact engagement in ball sports, and sustained attention to close work, such as reading. The eye skill that allows for binocular vision is called *vergence,* the ability to move both eyes simultaneously.

Here is how the other visual skills are categorized:

Eye Movement Control		
Name	**Definition**	**Impact**
Fixation	Ability to focus on a spot long enough to comprehend what you are looking at	Difficulty concentrating with activities such as reading
Saccadic	Ability of eyes to move accurately and smoothly from one object to another	Slow reader, loses place while reading, needs to re-read
Focusing near to far	Ability to quickly change focus from near to far to near automatically	Difficulty copying from a book, chalkboard, or overhead projector
Eye tracking	Ability to move the eyes while following or locating a moving object or to track a stationary object while moving	Loses place while reading, difficulty copying from the board, is a slow reader

Visual Perceptual Skills		
Name	**Definition**	**Impact**
Visual discrimination, visual foreground, visual figure ground	Ability to discriminate visual likeness and difference, figure-ground from foreground; visual closure (fill in visual information)	Reverse words or letters; poor discrimination with similar words or shapes; usually slow readers
Visual memory	Ability to visually recall past information	Lack of reading comprehension, may require an auditory cue to remember past visual information
Visualization	Ability to take the visual information that you already know and use it to project into the future a new visual scenario	Difficulty with spelling, math problems that deviate from specific learned skill; cannot project attaining future goals

Visual Motor Control		
Name	**Definition**	**Impact**
Visual gross motor	Ability to take in information and move the body based on that information (navigating around furniture in a room)	Extreme uneasiness in new environments and when things are moving around you; clumsiness; general insecurity with body movements that rely on visual cueing
Visual fine motor	Ability to take in information and move the hands based on that information (writing)	Handwriting difficulties; not able to copy patterns or difficulty with art projects

Q. How does the auditory system work?

A. Sound (vibrations of air) is received by the outer ear and travels to the ear drum, where it enters the middle ear. It is passed along the ossicular chain (comprised of the small bones in the middle ear), stimulating the fluid in the semicircular canal as it enters the inner ear and moves through cochlea. Finally, the sound is transformed into an electrical impulse that is carried by the cochlear nerve through the brain stem to the cortex.

Q. What are the common signs of auditory processing difficulties?

A. Here are some common challenges you may see in a child with auditory processing difficulties:

- Too sensitive to unexpected sounds
- Overly sensitive to loud noises
- Inattentive when spoken to
- Needs things repeated often
- Unable to pay attention when there is background noise
- Often misunderstands/confuses words that sound similar
- Slow responses during conversation

- Overly sensitive to certain sounds/voices
- Is not able to discern different sounds, such as fire alarm from class bell
- Misjudges distance of sounds; for example the sound of a train appears much closer

Q. What is the gustatory system and how does it work?

A. The gustatory system is our sense of taste. The gustatory receptors detect five main tastes: salty, sour, bitter, sweet, and savory. Interestingly, our brains register tastes as pleasurable or repulsive depending on how they are linked to our survival. If something we put into our mouths is essential for survival, the brain usually registers the taste chemical as pleasurable. If in some way, something we put on our tongue may be dangerous or make us sick, the brain registers it as displeasurable.

Your sensory perception of flavor is a team effort that involves your gustatory, somatosensory, and olfactory senses working together to create the taste experience. The gustatory qualities (salty, sour, bitter, sweet, and savory) arise from stimulation of taste receptors on the tongue. Somatosensory qualities arise from thermal, movement, and touch receptors on the tongue. Olfactory (smell) molecules that arise from flavors reach the olfactory epithelium through the back of the mouth and help us distinguish tastes.

Q. What is the olfactory sense and how does it work?

A. The olfactory sense is our sense of smell. The nose contains receptors that detect the chemicals around us and turn that information into electrical impulses. These impulses travel the olfactory nerve to the part of the brain responsible for detecting and decoding that information, the olfactory bulb. This area of the brain works with the limbic system (the emotional and memory center of the brain) to decode chemical information and attach meaning to it. The decoded chemical information is then checked against the stored knowledge of chemicals, allowing us to perceive a smell and attach emotional meaning to it. For example, the smell of bacon may remind you of Sunday mornings growing up, whereas the smell of exhaust may remind you of going to work.

The olfactory bulb is one of the few parts of the human brain where cells continue to regenerate from birth to death, which makes smell a lifetime memory reminder.

Q. What are common signs of olfactory/gustatory difficulties?

A. Here is a checklist of common difficulties with olfactory/gustatory system:

- Prefers either very bland or very spicy foods
- Is overly sensitive to smells (body odor, chemicals, etc.)
- Is overly focused on tastes and smells
- Picky eater

Chapter 3

RECOGNIZING SPD

- Does SPD impact my child's ability to engage in play activities?
- Why does my child refuse to play on playground equipment?
- Why can't my child figure out how to play with a new toy?
- Why can't my child play in a group situation?
- When someone throws a ball to my child, he covers his face and ducks. Why?
- Why does my teenager follow us around instead of doing something?
- Does SPD impact my child's academic performance?
- If my child is a slow reader, could this be linked to sensory processing difficulties?
- My child's teacher says she is smart but lazy. Could this be linked to SPD?
- Why is my "A" student flunking art?
- Are problems with handwriting a sign of SPD?
- Do sensory processing difficulties affect a child's social skills?
- Why does my child run in circles during recess rather than play with friends?
- Is purposely running into other children a sign of sensory difficulties?
- Why does my child avoid eye contact and seem socially awkward?
- Isn't it hard to separate behavior from sensory processing?
- If my child is accused of being purposefully disruptive at school, can it be SPD?
- My kindergartener hides after a few hours at school. Could this be due to SPD?
- Why can't my child sit still in school?
- Why does my child lie on the desk during school?
- Why do occupational therapists talk about bilateral coordination and crossing midline?
- Why are fine motor skills so important?

Q. Does SPD impact my child's ability to engage in play activities?

A. Yes. Children with SPD may have difficulties with a number of different aspects of play. Because of the dynamic nature of play, your child's nervous system is constantly taking in new information while referencing stored skill information. Play relies on effective sensory processing of visual and auditory information, as well as information from the primary senses (vestibular, proprioceptive, tactile), which are all crucial for environmental and interpersonal interactions. This is why play is so touted by developmental experts as crucial for early healthy development of the brain and body.

Q. Why does my child refuse to play on playground equipment?

A. Your child may be experiencing gravitational insecurity, which is one of the signs of vestibular processing difficulties. Since the vestibular sense (balance and motion sense) is crucial to developing a sense of physical security, children with vestibular difficulties are often fearful when their feet are off the ground, when their head position changes, or when they experience uncontrolled movement. Although many children go through periods in their development when they are more fearful of certain types of movement, it usually goes away fairly quickly. If this reaction continues and interferes with your child's ability to participate in age-appropriate activities, then you may need to seek help.

Here are some signs that a child may have gravitational insecurities:

- Extreme anxiety when feet leave the ground
- Does not like having his head upside down (parents may see this early)
- Unusual fear of heights or falling

- Uneasiness when walking on uneven surfaces or on stairs (may even appear dizzy)
- Extreme alarm when tipped backward, even with support

Q. Why can't my child figure out how to play with a new toy?

A. If your child is having sensory processing difficulties, this may impact his motor planning abilities, which help him figure out how to proceed. Most children figure out how to play with a new toy by experimenting and remembering how they used a similar toy in the past. However, children with motor planning difficulties struggle with how to plan the use of their fingers or body with a new toy. You can help your child by physically demonstrating how to do something new and letting him watch you repeat it over and over. Also, try breaking an activity down to smaller steps so that your child's brain doesn't have to motor plan an intricate series of actions, but rather smaller actions that will eventually come together for a complete activity. One of the best ways to do this for young children is by using pictures or a picture schedule so they see what to do first and then next.

Q. Why can't my child play in a group situation?

A. Think about yourself in a group situation. If you have ever thought about how much you have to concentrate in a group situation, it is staggering. Now try layering on top of that learning how to participate in a new activity. Interacting with people, as well as new activities, takes a tremendous amount of discerning attention to the outside world. A child must have her internal processing under control in order to move seamlessly in a very complicated situation.

You can help your child by starting her off in small organized group activities, often offered at therapy clinics or camps in the summer, or at local community centers. Organize a once-per-week semi-structured group time. Start with one other person and progress as your child seems more comfortable. Set up activities that alternate between little interaction with the others but a lot of input to the body, and other activities that provide more personal integration with light physical activity. For example, if your daughter and a couple of friends are playing Barbies or a board game, be sure you prompt a "jump on the trampoline" break every twenty or thirty minutes or when you suspect your daughter is becoming too overwhelmed by the intense social engagement.

Q. When someone throws a ball to my child, he covers his face and ducks. Why?

A. This is not uncommon for children who have visual/vestibular processing difficulties. The visual system allows us to see and discriminate information about objects but also allows us to judge the distance an object is from us, as well as the distance objects are from each other. In order to judge the distance of an object from you, you need to have a "sense" of where you are, which comes from your vestibular system. Your visual system, working with your vestibular system, allows you to visually track a moving object and determine its speed. If these systems are not working properly and communicating with each other, your child may not be able to judge where the ball is or how fast it is coming toward him, so you can imagine the panic he feels from an approaching ball.

Q. Why does my teenager follow us around instead of doing something?

A. Most kids welcome free time. However, children who have sensory processing disorder have a difficult time even thinking about what to do in the next five minutes, let alone making a weekend plan for activities. This is because children with sensory processing difficulties have difficulty projecting themselves into future situations. Often this points to vestibular difficulties since it is the vestibular system that is your "you are here" marker. If your "you are here" marker is broken, then it is difficult to foresee the second part of that sentence, which can be "…and then you will be there." As adults we can experience this when we are frazzled or overwhelmed. Sometimes it is difficult to determine what we should do next, even when we have a list of tasks to accomplish.

Q. Does SPD impact my child's academic performance?

A. Effective sensory processing sets the stage for more integrated skills, such as those required to be successful in school. When the sensory system is functioning properly, we receive, screen out, attend, process, and respond to sensory information in a useful way. If there is a breakdown in the process, it can impact the ability to learn. If your child is having difficulty with sensory processing, then it is likely to impact all aspects of his academic performance.

Q. If my child is a slow reader, could this be linked to sensory processing difficulties?

A. Yes, slow reading can be linked to difficulties with visual and/or vestibular processing. Because your vestibular system (balance and motion sense) controls the small muscles of the eyes, any difficulties with vestibular integration can have a significant impact on visual skills. Difficulty with eye teaming is one of the most common visual skill difficulties seen in school-aged children. Eye movement control skills also greatly affect reading comprehension and speed.

Here are some signs that visual skill difficulties are impacting a child's ability to read:

- Moves head while reading
- Skips phrases unknowingly
- Poor comprehension
- Covers one eye while reading (strongly indicates eye teaming difficulties)
- Complains that the text blurs or letters jump on the page

Note: If your child exhibits any of these difficulties, see a developmental optometrist. Your child's occupational therapist may be able to refer you to one.

Q. My child's teacher says she is smart but lazy. Could this be linked to SPD?

A. Children can be tired, overwhelmed, or bored, but in general their nervous systems are geared toward "discovering" the next thing, whether it be a new creature in their backyard or a new book. There may be something more going on with your child, and I encourage you to contact your child's pediatrician as well as the school occupational therapist for a screening. You and your child's teacher should fill out a sensory questionnaire to make sure you are seeing the same things at home and at school. This will help the professionals cluster behaviors to point you in the right direction.

Q. Why is my "A" student flunking art?

A. If a child has any tactile defensiveness, art class may seem more like torture class, especially if his art teacher is unaware of this difficulty. Can you imagine being tactically defensive and being asked to do papier-mâché—dip small strips of newspaper into a gooey glue solution and gently place them onto a model—or finger paint?

In addition, many children with SPD who have motor planning difficulties don't know how to make their imaginations come to life. They have trouble visualizing how something could look when finished and then making a plan to transform a mound of clay into a golden retriever.

If your child is tactically defensive, let his art teacher know. Suggest alternative activities that will give him deep-pressure input, such as working with heavy clay rather than doing a papier-mâché project. If your child has a motor planning difficulty, ask the art teacher if she could write down the steps for the project on a piece of paper.

Q. Are problems with handwriting a sign of SPD?

A. Difficulties with handwriting skills can have many causes. In boys, visual-motor skills as well as the neurons in the tips of the fingers develop later than in girls. This is the reason girls usually have superior fine motor skills early in life. So your child's difficulty could simply be due to timing, rather than an underlying neurological or sensory issue.

That said, handwriting struggles can be related to SPD. If your child displays difficulties with other fine motor activities, his hand appears weak, or he doesn't seem to know how much pressure to use on a pencil, he could be struggling with processing proprioceptive and tactile information. If he has difficulties copying simple shapes or patterns, he could be struggling with visual-motor integration. Observe your child in the classroom and look at the following things:

- How does he hold a pencil? Too light, too hard, or just right?
- How is his posture when he is writing? Is he lying on the desk or sitting upright?

- When he copies something, does he get lost on the page?
- Does he bounce in his seat, unable to focus on a fine motor task?

Q. Do sensory processing difficulties affect a child's social skills?

A. Absolutely! Social interactions are just about the most complicated sensory activity for humans. True social effectiveness relies on the ability of the nervous system to process all the said and unsaid information, interpret it, and then—in seconds—act on it. In addition to learned social skills, such as introducing yourself or looking at people when they speak, you must integrate what they are verbally and physically telling you, as well as be cognizant of anyone else that is part of the mix. If your child is having sensory processing issues, she is probably overwhelmed by all the sensory stimuli and as a result, she may shut down or appear inappropriate in social situations.

Q. Why does my child run in circles during recess rather than play with friends?

A. There are several SPD-related reasons for this behavior. Your child may have sat in a classroom for hours, trying to absorb and make sense of all the information around him, in some ways fighting to "keep it together" so he could learn and socially engage. Recess may be a time for him to regroup. Some children will spend the entire recess swinging or running in circles as a sensory integration strategy for calming and centering themselves. Or, your child may be fine in the more regimented classroom environment, but not understand the implicit social rules on the playground, causing him to behave in unusual ways. If your son has motor difficulties, the thought of joining in a motor-movement-type game can be overwhelming and/or embarrassing, so running in circles allows him to escape the possibility of having to be embarrassed in a game of four-square.

After talking to your child and finding out if his desire is to interact with one or two people but he is not comfortable in a large-group setting, ask your child's teacher if there are a couple other students that are not integrating into the playground group. If so, suggest a recess alternative with two or three students who can get together and play board games along with movement breaks, even if that means running in place. This would allow your child to interact with others in a more controlled smaller group, and the movement breaks would ensure he's getting some motor activity.

Q. Is purposely running into other children a sign of sensory difficulties?

A. If your child is purposely running into other children and knocking them over, he may be a sensory-seeker. He could be running into other children purposefully to get proprioceptive input. He probably does not understand that others don't like that kind of input/play. Explain to your child that rough-and-tumble play may be what his body needs, but it hurts the other children's bodies and upsets them. Try to make the point that when you make your friends feel mad, they will not want to play with you. A social story may be a great way to do this. Make sure to incorporate enough time for rougher play at home, so your child will be less aggressive in social situations.

Q. Why does my child avoid eye contact and seem socially awkward?

A. For many children and some adults with SPD, it is difficult to listen to someone and look at them at the same time. The vestibular (balance), visual, and auditory systems work closely together, so if someone is having difficulty processing sensory information, they may need to "cut off" one channel so that they can concentrate on the other one.

A child with difficulties processing sensory information from social situations is perhaps the most taxing of all. These children require a unique blend of internal sensory processing and natural external steps. This can be very difficult, because social effectiveness is hard to practice, as there are seemingly dire consequences when you fail.

Here are some things to consider when helping a child with SPD become more socially at ease:

- Try not to be uncomfortable with your child's efforts to be social, even when they are not effective. Reward the effort because it is very difficult to take that kind of risk.
- Help your child become aware of his own sensory issues in social situations. Use programs such as "How Does Your Engine Run" and apply that to social situations.
- Consider putting your child on a sensory diet (described in Chapter 6) and have him do certain sensory activities that have a more calming effect right before a social event.
- Use social stories to help your child know how he should act in a given social situation.
- Try role play for upcoming social situations (older children really benefit from this). You can videotape your child role-playing and have her watch it so she can see herself socially engaging.

Q. Isn't it hard to separate behavior from sensory processing?

A. We cannot separate the two. A healthy sensory system is the foundation for productive behavior. Behavior encompasses many things that make us adaptable and successful in our environments, such as screening out irrelevant information to pay attention, attending to an activity for a sufficient amount of time, transitioning from one activity to another, following directions, moving attention from the big picture to the details and back again, as well as completing an activity once started.

Q. If my child is accused of being purposefully disruptive at school, can it be SPD?

A. Yes. Sensory processing difficulties can often manifest as difficulties such as not sitting still, falling out of the chair, throwing tantrums when faced with transitions, running around in circles when asked to perform fine motor tasks, or simply shutting down in different situations and disengaging when asked to perform a task. Many times these children will be described as disruptive, non-cooperative, impulsive, unwilling to listen, unable to sit still, or unwilling to work. It is important to observe how disruptive behavior is impacting the child and then group behaviors together to point to a possible underlying cause.

Even if your child's sensory defensiveness decreases, he may still misbehave. It is important to keep in mind that most children are not willful with their behaviors. There is usually a reason for a child's behavior, and sometimes it is simply a matter of finding out what motivates that child. Sometimes therapists and parents have to help a child "unlearn" a behavior learned as a result of reactions caused by sensory processing difficulties or even the environment. Your child's "misbehavior" may be a learned response to the reaction of fear brought on by the sensory defensiveness. Now that his sensory defensiveness has lessened, the learned behaviors may still be present and will have to be untaught.

Q. My kindergartener hides after a few hours at school. Could this be due to SPD?

A. Yes, it is likely that your child "holds it together" to be a part of the group for a few hours and then just becomes overwhelmed. Although kindergarten can be fun for a lot of children, those who have difficulty processing sensory information are easily overwhelmed in this sort of environment. There are two things at play here. First, your child is in a stimulating and demanding sensory environment with other children laughing, crying, running around, and playing (basically being kindergarteners), as well as teachers talking and directing activity. Second, there are many things in the room that are visually interesting. That adds up to quite a bit of visual and auditory stimulation, and on top of that, there are demands being placed on your child to follow directions and be part of a group. Your child may be overwhelmed, and hiding is his way of shutting down. The trick may be for the teacher to give him periodic breaks from stimulation throughout the day so his nervous system does not feel the need to completely shut down.

Q. Why can't my child sit still in school?

A. Today, schools offer very little opportunity for movement. All developing nervous systems crave movement, and a child who has difficulties processing sensory information may crave or need it even more. The other children sitting at their desks all day are also having a hard time sitting still, but they are able to convince their bodies to sit still. Your daughter may not be able to do that. Ask the teacher if your daughter can take "movement" breaks throughout the day. It would be great if you could convince her to let the whole class be on a movement schedule (suggest Brain Gym activities; see Chapter 16). If your daughter's teacher is reluctant to do either, ask if your daughter can be assigned some class chores that involve movement, such as passing out papers, moving chairs, running attendance to the front office, or sharpening pencils. Also, consider asking the school occupational therapist if your daughter can use a sensory cushion (this is a wedge or a circle cushion that has air in it), which provides slight movement that is usually not distracting.

Q. Why does my child lie on the desk during school?

A. If your child also slumps at the table at home or appears to be leaning against something while standing, exhibits a slumped posture in general, or tires more easily than his peers during physical activities and appears to have low tone in his muscles, he may have proprioceptive processing difficulties, often called postural disorder. His brain is not getting sufficient feedback from his joints and muscles about where his body is in relation to itself. After his teacher reminds him to sit up, he can probably sit up straight for a few minutes because he is thinking about it. As soon as someone calls his name or he has to pay attention to what the teacher is saying, he must use his cognitive energy elsewhere and so lies on his desk again. Because his nervous system is not doing its job in the background, he must consciously make his body do something most of us do naturally. Give your child a small visual reminder, such as a little picture of a child sitting upright at his desk, perhaps placed on the corner of his own desk. A good physical endurance program that provides a lot of proprioceptive input and challenges the muscles at the body's core can also help.

Q. Why do occupational therapists talk about bilateral coordination and crossing midline?

A. Together, bilateral coordination and crossing midline lay the foundation for gross and fine motor skills. Bilateral coordination is using both sides of the body to accomplish a task. A few examples are using both hands together to catch a ball or push a rolling pin. An example of the hands coordinating different actions to accomplish a task is stabilizing a jar with one hand and unscrewing it with the other, or pulling a button hole while you push the button through with the other hand.

Crossing midline is the act of traversing the center of the body with an arm, leg or eyes to perform an action on the opposite side of the body, such as kicking a soccer ball with your right leg across the left side of your body or putting an earring in your left ear with your right hand. We have to cross midline with our eyes when we read or scan across the room without moving our head.

Q. Why are fine motor skills so important?

A. Fine motor skills are everything you do with your hands, such as buttoning, belting, zipping/unzipping, screwing jar lids on/off, writing, using scissors to cut, putting makeup on, and typing. Fine motor skills are dependent on the development of gross motor skills in the early years. For example, the proprioceptive pressure a child gains while crawling helps develop the arches of the hands, which are crucial for balance, stability, and mobility in the hand. These capabilities allow us to write, use appropriate force to grip an object, and lift an object.

Chapter 4

OTHER SIGNS AND SYMPTOMS

- Why is my child so emotionally immature, compared to other children?
- Why does my child have a meltdown when his scheduled is changed?
- Why is my child scared of unexpected noises?
- Are motor skills affected by sensory processing disorder?
- Are poor balance skills a result of sensory processing difficulties?
- What is the W-seated position, and why do children with SPD prefer to sit this way?
- Is walking on tiptoes related to sensory issues?
- Is a speech delay a sign of SPD?
- What is verbal dyspraxia?
- What are some early signs of verbal dyspraxia?
- What are oral-motor difficulties?
- Is social communication related to sensory integration difficulties?

Q. Why is my child so emotionally immature, compared to other children?

A. There is a strong link between effective sensory processing and emotional control. When a child's sensory-nervous system is not processing the world around it accurately and automatically, the child is in a constant state of uncertainty. In some cases, this can be seen as emotional insecurity or instability. A child who has SPD is constantly trying to protect herself from the outside environment with a body that is not always supplying the child with correct information. Your daughter may be acting on some misinterpretation from her nervous system, leading her to act in a way that others perceive as emotionally immature.

Q. Why does my child have a meltdown when his scheduled is changed?

A. Try to imagine that you are driving a car in the dark and the lights just went out, but you know the road like the back of your hand and so you know you can make it home. Now imagine someone changed the road. You would either be stuck in a ditch or lost somewhere. How would you feel? Many children who have sensory processing difficulties rely on outside structure, whether it's a schedule set in stone or environmental cues. This structure provides a framework that your child knows how to navigate without having to worry about changes in the outside world. When the set schedule changes, he may not be able to see himself doing whatever the new thing is, because he had prepared his body and brain to do what was originally planned. To one child it may be seen as an exciting new activity, but to a child with SPD, it is like being pushed out on stage in front of a live audience without a script.

Q. Why is my child scared of unexpected noises?

A. Your child may have auditory defensiveness. She is reacting this way because she is processing unexpected sounds as very scary, irritating, or stressful. Some people with auditory defensiveness are only sensitive to certain sounds, such as sirens or vacuum cleaners. However, some children may be sensitive to everyday noises, such as fans, fluorescent lights, computers, water dripping from a faucet, or even the air conditioner.

Many children who have auditory defensiveness also have vestibular processing problems. These children will have difficulties localizing a sound, which increases their fears. For example, the sound of the vacuum cleaner may seem like it is surrounding them, instead of coming from one little machine.

Q. Are motor skills affected by sensory processing disorder?

A. Yes, praxis (motor planning) difficulties are one of the major reasons children are referred to occupational therapy in the schools. Effective motor planning relies on good balance, understanding where you are in space, having a sense of where your body is in relation to itself, as well as the ability to discriminate touch information. Locating and discriminating auditory information as well as visual information is also important for the brain in planning motor activities.

Motor planning (called "praxis" in the medical world) is the ability to plan and initiate a skilled act in sequence from beginning to end. Motor planning is the link between cognitive function and motor output, effectively connecting your brain to your muscles. It is considered one of the most complex functions for a developing nervous system.

If your child seems to be highly uncoordinated, she may be having motor planning difficulties. The first few times a child has to manipulate her body in a new environment, she has to consciously think about each and every motion. After she does it a few times, the action becomes automatic. She is able to navigate around desks, talk to her friends, and listen to the teacher at the same time. The child who has difficulty with motor planning must consciously think about how her body is going to interact with the environment. New skills are not easily moved from conscious control to automatic control, which may cause a lack of coordination. It is very difficult for anyone to consciously think about several things at once, thus it is essential that motor planning be intact so that everyday tasks are automatic. If you had to "think" about chewing gum while walking, you would either bite your tongue or trip!

Q. Are poor balance skills a result of sensory processing difficulties?

A. Balance problems can result from many different conditions, such as an ear infection, anatomical malformations, or sensory processing difficulties. Because good balance relies on three sensory systems working together (the visual system, the vestibular system, and the proprioceptive system), difficulties with any one of the systems can result in poor balance, especially when a child is engaged in activities that require movement.

Q. What is the W-seated position, and why do children with SPD prefer to sit this way?

A. The W-seated position, although not comfortable to most adults, provides a wide, stable base of support for children. Some children with SPD have low muscle tone, which points to difficulties in processing proprioceptive information. This impacts motor coordination and postural stability, and it takes a good deal of extra energy to maintain an unsupported seated position for these children.

Sitting in the W-seated position can excessively stretch out muscles and tendons around the hip and knee joints, which could eventually contribute to decreased balance while standing. Although it is very hard to stop a child from sitting in this position because it feels safer, you want to work with your child to try different seating options on the floor that provide some support and still allow her to play. Try a bean-bag chair, form a u-shape around your child using a rolled-up blanket for support, or encourage your child to lie on a pillow on her stomach when she gets tired. This position will still allow her to play and also continues to provide proprioceptive input to her upper extremity joints.

Q. Is walking on tiptoes related to sensory issues?

A. It is not uncommon for young children who are new to walking to walk on their toes initially. However, a consistent heel strike appears at about eighteen to twenty-two months old in most children. Many children who have SPD continue to walk on their toes beyond this age because it heightens their sensory input.

Children with hypersensitivity to touch may walk on their toes to limit the amount of tactile stimulation to their feet. Other children may stiffen their bodies in such a way that they are in a constant state of extension, bouncing on the balls of their feet and toes. There is also a condition referred to as idiopathic toe walking (ITW), in which children walk on their toes in the absence of any known cause. There is evidence that children who are chronic toe-walkers have a higher incidence of speech/language delays, fine motor, visual-motor, and gross motor delays. The bottom line is that consistent toe-walking past two years old should be brought to the attention of your child's pediatrician because it may be a sign of underlying problems.

Q. Is a speech delay a sign of SPD?

A. Yes, a speech delay may be the result of underlying sensory processing difficulties. Many aspects of neurological functioning impact our ability to communicate effectively. For instance, if a child is having auditory processing difficulties, he may have difficulty locating where sounds are coming from or discriminating between similar yet different sounds. This will impact his understanding of language as well as his expressive speech. If a child has tactile/proprioceptive processing difficulties, this could affect oral-motor skills. Using your lips, tongue, and other articulators correctly to form words is a very complicated oral-motor skill. In addition, many children with sensory processing difficulties have poor muscle tone, which may result in weak muscles around the jaw, cheeks, lips, and tongue. Tactile defensiveness can also interfere with a child's ability to use his mouth correctly, affecting speech production.

Q. What is verbal dyspraxia?

A. Verbal dyspraxia is a motor programming disorder that makes it difficult to execute and sequence voluntary motor movements of the small muscles of the mouth. These movements are required to produce speech as well as combine speech sounds to form syllables, words, phrases, and sentences in a controlled manner. Children with verbal dyspraxia hear and understand words, but cannot get all the small muscles of the mouth and tongue to move in a coordinated way. Sometimes they may be able to produce words or sounds when they are not thinking about it, but when asked to replicate the same word or sound again, they are unable to reproduce the sequence of oral-motor actions necessary to say the word.

Q. What are some early signs of verbal dyspraxia?

A. The following are some common early signs of verbal dyspraxia:

- Has difficulties with other fine motor skills
- Uses limited or little babbling as an infant (void of many consonants)—first words may appear late or not at all; pointing and "grunting" may be all that is heard

- Able to open and close mouth, lick lips, and protrude, retract, and lateralize tongue while eating, but not when directed to do so
- Has difficulty speaking on demand, even though speaking spontaneously is not a problem
- Displays continuous grunting and pointing beyond age two
- Shows limited use of consonants—child may only use b, m, p, t, d, and h
- Has difficulty combining consonants and vowels into words
- Is able to articulate simple words but will not use them purposefully in a sentence
- Appears to understand much more language than she can express
- One syllable or word is favored and used to convey all or many words beyond age two
- Speaks mostly in vowels
- Gets "stuck" on a previously uttered word, or brings oral-motor elements from a previous word into the next word uttered

Q. What are oral-motor difficulties?

A. A child with oral-motor difficulties may have trouble chewing, sucking, blowing, and/or making certain speech sounds. The child may have low muscle tone in the face ("long" or "droopy" face), a "flat affect" look, or open-mouth breathing.

Q. Is social communication related to sensory integration difficulties?

A. Sensory processing difficulties will directly affect social communication. This is because social communication requires attending to incoming sensory stimuli from others, such as body language, auditory and visual input, as well as the greater environment.

Chapter 5

GETTING A DIAGNOSIS

- Who should treat my child with SPD?
- What else should I consider when looking for an occupational therapist?
- Does the occupational therapist's personality really matter?
- What questions should I ask the occupational therapist?
- What should I tell the OT about my child?
- Are there tests that can determine if my child has sensory issues?
- Is it difficult to get school-based occupational therapy for SPD?
- Is therapy received in a clinic different from therapy received in a school?
- Should I stop occupational therapy if my child's behavior becomes worse?
- What information do I need to give the OT about my child's behavior?
- If I don't see any changes after three months of OT, what should I do?
- What if I can't afford weekly occupational therapy sessions?
- If my child has SPD but he's not in special education, how can I get help from his school?
- Will my insurance company pay for sensory integration therapy?
- How do I get a prescription for occupational therapy?
- What if the doctor gives my child a diagnosis that is not related to SPD?
- How long does occupational therapy usually last?
- How much does occupational therapy for sensory integration cost?
- How do I know if my two-year-old requires early intervention services?

Q. Who should treat my child with SPD?

A. Working with children with sensory processing difficulties is primarily the domain of occupational therapists (OTs). The occupational therapy curriculum consists of core courses in the areas of neurology, gross anatomy, physiology, and courses that teach how to break down everyday tasks (such as dressing) into the sequential neuro-motor steps required for that task. Occupational therapy schools offer pediatric-specific courses that teach sensory integration theory and application, as well as other theory applications, such as neuro-developmental therapy. Occupational therapists can be thought of as the ambassadors of the nervous system. An OT can evaluate the link between your child's nervous system and the function or "occupation" of being a child, such as learning and playing.

Occupational therapists work in many different areas, such as hand therapy, geriatrics, mental health, and pediatrics. You want to contact a pediatric occupational therapist who has experience working with children with SPD. Occupational therapists who are "SIPT certified" have had advanced training in sensory integration theory, testing, and treatment, specifically the sensory integration praxis test. However, many pediatric occupational therapists are quite knowledgeable about how to diagnose and treat kids with SPD even though they are not "certified." The best thing you can do is have a conversation with the OT and inquire about his or her experience working with SPD. It is also very important that the OT you choose believes in working closely with your family and the other professionals that are involved in your child's life. This will guarantee more effective embedding of treatment in every aspect of your child's life.

Q. What else should I consider when looking for an occupational therapist?

A. The considerations are similar to what you would look for when choosing a pediatrician or even a preschool.

- What is the personality and energy level of the therapist?
- Where is the clinic located? Is it close to your home, work, and/or your child's school?
- What hours is the therapist available to work with your child?
- Will the therapy schedule work with your child's school schedule?

Q. Does the occupational therapist's personality really matter?

A. You want to make sure your child meshes with the occupational therapist's personality and energy level. Some children respond better to "over-the-top," high-energy people, whereas other children feel safer and respond better to a more "low-key" person. Most occupational therapists working with children know how to gear their energy levels to fit the child. Some other things to consider include the following: How open is the therapist to questions? If your child has dual households, how comfortable does the therapist seem in making sure everyone is included in the therapy? Is the therapist willing to have the parents or caregiver present during some sessions so you can learn how to help your child? The bottom line is to take the time to have a discussion with the potential therapist to see if it is a good fit.

Q. What questions should I ask the occupational therapist?

A. The following questions help set the stage for what you deem as important in a therapist, and they will make your therapist aware of your needs up front.

- Why did you choose to work in pediatrics? (This should give you a sense of the occupational therapist's passion and commitment.)
- How long have you been working in pediatrics?
- Have you treated many children with Sensory Processing Disorder?
- Can you tell me some of the different types of sensory processing difficulties you have worked with?
- Do you have advanced training in sensory integration?
- What is your policy on "family training" and communication?
- Will you communicate with other members of my child's team?

A friendly note: Make sure you ask these questions in a friendly way, because you want your OT to desire to work with you and your family.

Q. What should I tell the OT about my child?

A. The occupational therapist will probably have you fill out a questionnaire related to your child's history and current issues. Questions concerning birth history, developmental milestones, behavior issues, and speech development should be addressed. If there is something significant that the questionnaire doesn't cover, include it with the paperwork and mention it to your therapist, so the therapist can consider everything during your child's evaluation. Make sure to let your child's therapist know of any family history that may be pertinent, especially any neurological or mental diagnoses in either parent's family history. Also, you should talk to your parents and your spouse's parents to see if you or your spouse had any sensory type behaviors as children.

Q. Are there tests that can determine if my child has sensory issues?

A. There are a number of tests an occupational therapist may employ in order to determine your child's sensory involvement. The most powerful evaluative tools are the reports of family members and teachers, along with clinical observations of your child in action. Some formal evaluations that a therapist can use are:

- Sensory Integration Praxis Test (SIPT). Designed to assess the state of sensory integration and praxis for children ages four to eight years old. It gives very detailed, quantifiable information. A therapist must be certified to administer the SIPT.
- Sensory Profile by Winnie Dunn. Uses a questionnaire format to categorize observable behaviors. There are four versions: Infant/Toddler Sensory Profile (0–3 years), Sensory Profile (3–10 years), Adolescent/Adult Sensory Profile (11 and up), and Sensory Profile School Companion (3–11 years).
- Sensory Processing Measure. Designed to give a complete characterization of a child's sensory functions by looking at the child in three environments: home, main classroom, and school environment.
- Simple checklists can also be very useful. One that is used often with educators is the preschool checklist contained in *Answers to Questions Teachers Ask about Sensory Integration* by Carol Kranowitz.
- Bruininks-Oseretsky Test of Motor Proficiency. This test is designed to test the motor capabilities of children. It can be used with children who are able-bodied, children who have dyspraxia, as well as those with developmental delays. It is applicable for ages four to twenty-two years.
- Peabody Developmental Motor Scales

- The Carolina Curriculum. This is an assessment and intervention tool for use with children birth to five.
- Developmental Test of Visual Perception (DTVP)
- Test of Visual Motor Skills
- Beery-Buktenica Developmental Test of Visual Motor Integration (VMI)
- Miller Function and Participation Scales
- The Quick Neurological Screening Test (QNST)
- ETCH Handwriting Assessment. The assessment may include various handwriting tests.
- SCERTS Model/Assessment. Designed for children with autism, this evaluation is best completed with a team.

Note: These are just some of the tests available to occupational therapists. Your child's therapist may use different assessment tools.

Q. Is it is difficult to get school-based occupational therapy for SPD?

A. This depends on the school district and the sensory processing awareness level of the special education team. Occupational therapists in the schools have to consider the educational relevancy for therapy and must always make sure the occupational therapy goals for your child support his academic goals. Some schools are reluctant to allow occupational therapists to assess a child for sensory processing disorder, especially if the child has not already been identified as needing other special education services. One of the keys is not to ask for a sensory processing evaluation but to ask for an occupational therapy evaluation based on difficulties your child is having with accessing the educational curriculum or the educational environment.

Q. Is therapy received in a clinic different from therapy received in a school?

A. If your child's school has a sensory gym, the treatment will be very similar to the setup in an occupational therapy clinic designed to address sensory needs.

However, most schools do not have sensory gyms. Many times, school-based occupational therapists don't have access to vestibular equipment (swinging equipment), which is crucial when treating children with sensory processing difficulties. However, most school-based occupational therapists become skilled at adapting the environment for treatment or designing activities to challenge your child. These treatment activities work on the sensory as well as motor difficulties that may be impacting your child's academics, and many of them will be embedded throughout his day.

You want the OT to work closely with the classroom teacher, PE teacher, and others who interact with your child so that the OT has increased understanding of your child's sensory needs and can utilize some of the suggested sensory strategies. To get more involved in your child's therapy at school, call or leave a note for your child's occupational therapist to set up a time to talk. Tell the OT you want to be updated periodically on your child's therapy (email updates usually work well). Ask for some activities you can do at home to help your child.

Q. Should I stop occupational therapy if my child's behavior becomes worse?

A. It is very common for children who have SPD to "lose it" when they first begin a new therapy program. The therapist is asking your child to engage in activities that challenge her nervous system, which may be overwhelming. It is hard for any of us to get out of our comfort zone, much less a child who has been battling her own nervous system for years. Keep in mind that she is engaging in therapy in a safe environment, and this will eventually help your daughter to take in the information and make sense of it in her everyday life. Make the therapist aware of your daughter's behavior and remember that sensory integration therapy is a slow but steady process.

Q. What information do I need to give the OT about my child's behavior?

A. It is important to let the occupational therapist know about changes you are seeing at home and any concerns you have. It is a good idea to keep records of the changes, to note when they are occurring, time of day, if they precede or follow a certain event, as well as how long the behavior lasts. Also, when you record the behavior, be sure to use objective descriptions such as "dropped to the floor and pounded the floor" or "ran to the corner and cried" rather than something like, "threw a fit." This information will help the occupational therapist tailor the treatment in the clinic, as well as provide you with some in-home strategies.

Q. If I don't see any changes after three months of OT, what should I do?

A. Here's a rule of thumb that many therapists hold to: if no positive changes are seen after six weeks of therapy, therapy needs to change. In most cases, you should see a difference within a month or two of therapy, sometimes in a week. The changes vary depending on the severity of the issue, the age of the child, and the amount of "protective armor" the nervous system has already built up.

It's time to talk to your child's therapist and ask some questions. First, what changes is she seeing in the clinic or school setting? Second, ask the therapist what her short-term and long-term goals are. Third, ask to have a list of activities that she is working on and information about how you can adapt them at home to have a greater impact on your child's success.

Q. What if I can't afford weekly occupational therapy sessions?

A. First, make sure you thoroughly understand the occupational therapist's evaluation. Get clarification about the specific sensory processing areas where your child is struggling most and how sensory processing disorder is affecting his life. Explain to the therapist that you are not able to afford therapy right now but want strategies so that you can start helping your child at home and school. Second, call the special education director at your school and explain the recent OT evaluation. Request a school-based occupational therapy evaluation. Remember, in order to qualify for educationally based occupational therapy, the difficulties must impact the child's ability to participate in his educational environment.

Q. If my child has SPD but he's not in special education, how can I get help from his school?

A. First, request a teacher conference and explain your child's difficulties to the teacher. Explain how these difficulties may impact your child in the classroom. This is very important because most teachers want to help the kids they teach and respond well once they understand that a child requires specific intervention to access the curriculum the teacher is presenting. If your child continues to struggle in the classroom, request a meeting with your child's teacher, principal, and the school's resource teacher so that you can get a team of people together to help solve the issue. A new federal mandate in place called Response to Intervention (RTI) requires schools to meet the needs of students who are struggling but not in special education. The school will examine the child's classroom environment and look for ways it can be slightly adapted before initiating special education services.

Q. Will my insurance company pay for sensory integration therapy?

A. Insurance coverage for sensory integration therapy is hit or miss. If you suspect your child has SPD or have already been told by an occupational therapist that your child requires therapy, take some steps to increase the chances of insurance coverage.

- Get a doctor's order for the specific types of occupational therapy your child needs.
- Call your insurance company and ask if it covers occupational therapy.
- Make sure that you ask if there are any exceptions to this coverage. Some exclusions may include:
  - Diagnoses that are related to a developmental delay
  - Diagnoses that appear to be educationally related
  - Therapy unrelated to injury or congenital condition
- Ask how many visits per year the company will approve.
- Ask what diagnostic and CPT codes are covered.

Here is some smart consumer advice to use when dealing with insurance companies:

- Make sure you record the time and date anytime you have a discussion about coverage with your insurance carrier.
- Always ask for the name of your representative and how you can get in touch with that person again.

- Know that just because a representative gave you a quote of benefits over the phone, this is no guarantee of coverage.
- Make sure you know what your deductible and out-of-pocket expenses are, as well as the percentage of coverage once the deductible is met.
- Ask for confirmation by repeating back what the insurance representative has told you.

Most therapy clinics have an *insurance reimbursement* option in which you pay first and then turn your bill in to your insurance company for reimbursement. Before you take this route, make sure you know all the requirements from your insurance company to get reimbursement and make sure you pass on this information to the therapy clinic. The clinic will likely agree to attach the requirements to the bill so you can pursue reimbursement. Keep in mind that the amount each insurance company will reimburse does vary. This is something you want to find out first. Also, the therapy clinic may provide a discount for cash payments since they don't have to spend the time billing insurance. Make sure you ask about this before beginning treatment.

Q. How do I get a prescription for occupational therapy?

A. Call a pediatric OT clinic and explain what your suspicions are and ask if they will do a "quick screener" on your child. Explain to the therapist that you simply want a short overview description of your child's difficulties. The OT can do this by having you fill out a sensory checklist and then seeing your child briefly. Based on this information, the OT can write a justification for further in-depth evaluation and treatment, if necessary. This makes getting a doctor's prescription for treatment much easier.

Q. What if the doctor gives my child a diagnosis that is not related to SPD?

A. You may believe the underlying issues are sensory but may receive a diagnosis of something different. Tell your doctor your concerns and the research you have done prior to the appointment. When you describe your child's difficulties, try not to use diagnostic labels. You want the doctor to make an accurate diagnosis based on your description of your child's behaviors. If you feel that the behaviors you are seeing are interfering with your child's daily life, make sure your doctor understands that waiting to see if your child outgrows these behaviors is not an option.

Ask yourself if you are comfortable with your child receiving a diagnostic label. This is hard because this diagnostic label may not be what you believe your child has, but it also may be the quickest road to getting him services through the insurance company.

If the doctor doesn't agree that your child has sensory processing difficulties, you may want to obtain a sensory checklist yourself and fill it out. Bring that to your child's doctor appointment. Sometimes seeing the symptoms on paper helps a physician make a diagnosis. If your doctor appears reluctant to pursue your concerns further, you may have to ask for a second opinion. Call a pediatric therapy clinic that specializes in sensory integration and ask if they can recommend a pediatrician in the area who is knowledgeable about sensory integration and occupational therapy.

Q. How long does occupational therapy usually last?

A. This will vary greatly. Some children receive occupational therapy for a few months and with a continuing home program appear "good-to-go." Other children may have to attend therapy for a few years. The best estimate will come from your child's occupational therapist after seeing how your child responds to therapy. Some of this will be dependent on other diagnoses, as well as a family's willingness and time to carry out therapeutic strategies.

The doctor's prescription or insurance carrier may dictate the length and extent of your child's therapy. A doctor's prescription will read something like, "occupational therapy two times per week for ten weeks." Following a comprehensive occupational therapy evaluation that consists of sensory integration and praxis testing, your child's therapist will be able to give you an idea of how much therapy is necessary and how long your child should participate. The therapist may even call the doctor's office and ask for more time.

Keep in mind that your therapist will reevaluate your child's progress regularly and suggest continuing or discontinuing therapy, based on the level of progress.

Q. How much does occupational therapy for sensory integration cost?

A. The price for therapy is dependent upon where you live. Prices can range from $90 per hour session to $200 per hour session, averaging around $140 to $165 per hour, with some discounts given to individuals who pre-pay cash.

Q. How do I know if my two-year-old requires early intervention services?

A. There is no exact rule of thumb, but if you feel your child is not developing normally or is delayed in reaching several milestones, bring this to the attention of your pediatrician. The following are some indicators that you should pursue an evaluation by an early intervention therapist.

Note: Every child reaches milestones at different ages, and there is a range in what is considered normal/typical development.

Gross Motor

- Not sitting upright by one year
- Not standing unaccompanied by fourteen months
- Not walking by eighteen months
- Walking on toes, not soles of feet
- Falls frequently for no observable reason

Fine Motor

- Uses a fisted grasp on a crayon
- Not able to copy simple lines and a circle by age four
- Displays uncoordinated movements during activities
- Uses one hand to participate in activities
- Does not exhibit a hand preference by age four

Sensory

- Afraid of swinging movements; does not like to be upside down
- Over/underreactive to pain
- Has difficulty calming down appropriately
- Touches everything—including people, objects
- Avoids messy projects and does not like to touch
- Lack of eye contact
- Hyper/hypotonic (rigid or floppy muscle tone)
- Does not appear to hear sounds or people's voices

Social/Behavior

- Does not display joint attention (wants others to pay attention to what she is attending to)

- Does not copy actions of others by age two
- Does not exhibit pretend play by age two
- Does not demonstrate typical play with toys
- Is overly fixated on a limited repertoire of activities (this can be typical in normal development, but abnormal fixation interferes with social interaction or other activities during the day)

Eating/Speech

- Silent; doesn't babble or try to imitate sounds as an infant
- Difficulty biting/chewing food
- Does not initiate feeding self by one and a half years
- Not able to drink from a cup at one and a half years
- Lack of early babbling
- Is not gaining words by age two

Chapter 6

TREATMENT

- Is there medication for SPD?
- What is sensory integration therapy?
- Is there a standard treatment regime I can follow for my child?
- What is a sensory diet?
- Can I use a sensory diet designed for one child with another child who also has sensory needs?
- Should I give my child's home sensory diet to her teacher?
- Are there different types of sensory diets?
- What is the best therapy for a child just diagnosed with SPD?
- My child's therapy sessions look like play to me. What am I paying for?
- Are mixed play groups beneficial to children with SPD?
- Would a mixed preschool designed for high-functioning autistic children be beneficial to a child with SPD?
- What is a "brushing program"?
- What is Therapeutic Listening?
- What is the Listening Program, and how is it different from Therapeutic Listening?
- What about Auditory Integration Training?
- Is all therapy weekly or biweekly, or are other types of therapy available?
- What is intensive therapy?
- Are there camps devoted to working on sensory integration difficulties?
- Are there other types of therapy besides occupational therapy?

Q. Is there medication for SPD?

A. Yes, but the medication does not come in a bottle. Rather, it can be embedded into your child's everyday life. The hard news is that it will not change your child quickly. Interventions for sensory processing disorder may take years and will definitely take the work of all those involved in the child's life.

Q. What is sensory integration therapy?

A. Early sensory integration therapy concentrated on providing a child with tactile, proprioceptive, and vestibular input to enhance and/or counter how the child's nervous system processes the information from these senses. Research and some tenacious therapists pushed sensory integration therapy to also include interventions that enhance auditory and visual processing. A large component of therapy is helping a child to better understand how the sensory-nervous systems impact behavior and perceptions as well as how to cope with sensory processing difficulties.

Q. Is there a standard treatment regime I can follow for my child?

A. There is no standard program for treatment intervention. Your child has different strengths and deficits than the next child with sensory processing difficulties. Furthermore, the characteristics manifest themselves in varying degrees in each child's life. Treatment for sensory integration must be designed to address the individual needs of a child, first taking into account how the sensory processing difficulties are impacting that child's daily life. Before designing interventions, a therapist will consider your child's age and cognitive abilities, as well as the support system at home and at school.

Q. What is a sensory diet?

A. A sensory diet is an individualized program of sensory activities designed to help a specific child function better at home and school. This program should be set up and monitored by an occupational therapist who is familiar with your child's sensory needs. It is important to remember the program that works today may not be the same one that will work three months from now. The program will be modified to meet your child's changing needs.

Usually, a sensory diet is designed by the occupational therapist in conjunction with the family and other team members. A sensory diet will not be successful if it is carried out only during occupational therapy sessions. The sensory diet activities must be implemented by the family and every one else on the team.

Frankly, all children would probably benefit from a sensory diet. Many of today's children get bombarded with too much of one kind of sensation and too little of other kinds. A sensory diet is simply a way for your child to get a well-balanced set of activities to reach an optimal level of engagement in her surroundings. A child who has sensory processing disorder requires a sensory diet. It helps a child with modulation difficulties to react appropriately by learning self-regulation strategies; it increases the focus of a child by helping her engage in activities that calm overarousal; and it increases the activity level of an underaroused child.

Activities such as dance can also play a positive role if they get your child active and engaged. Some of these activities may even be a part of a sensory diet, but for a child who has sensory processing difficulties, it is important to have specific sensory activities infused into her day.

Q. Can I use the same sensory diet designed for one child with another child who also displays sensory needs?

A. It is important that sensory diets be individualized, because each child processes information differently and requires different types of sensory input to engage in the world. However, it does not hurt for you to try different techniques that worked for one child on another child. Just make sure you pay attention to the different reactions and consult your child's therapist.

Q. Should I give my child's home sensory diet to her teacher?

A. Typically, sensory diets designed for the home environment need to be modified for the school environment. Your daughter's teacher could feel overwhelmed by all of the sensory diet activities and not know where to begin. Make sure the school occupational therapist has a copy of your child's home sensory diet. If your child is not seeing an occupational therapist at school, ask her private occupational therapist to suggest some sensory diet activities that could be infused into the school day. It is important to be sensitive to the fact that the teacher has a whole class of students, so ask your child's therapist to suggest activities that the whole class can engage in or at least that are not disruptive to the others in the class.

Q. Are there different types of sensory diets?

A. Each sensory diet is different in that it is tailored for the specific needs of each child. Here is a brief example of what a sensory diet may look like:

Sensory Diet

Date _____   Name _____

School _____   Age _____

Time	Key Events in the Day	Support Sensory Diet Activities	Comment / Sign Off

_____
OT Signature

_____
Teacher Signature

Keep in mind that sensory diet activities are tailored specifically to meet the needs of individual children. Here are a few common activities for home and school designed to work on specific sensory issues.

Sensory diet for home
Vestibular—roll down a hill, spin in a chair, sit-n-spin
Proprioceptive—vacuum, carry laundry, jump on trampoline, pillow crashing, roll child in blanket
Tactile—play with Play-Doh, find objects in rice bins
Auditory—listen to therapeutic CDs
Visual—ball activities with varying sizes and colors of balls

Sensory diet for school
Vestibular—use playground swings, monkey bars (upside down)
Proprioceptive—carry books, play hopscotch
Tactile—use squeeze toys (e.g., balls with tentacles, etc.)
Auditory—engage in Therapeutic Listening or Metronome
Visual—place a three-folder "wall" on the desk to reduce overstimulation and visual distraction during tests

Q. What is the best therapy for a child just diagnosed with SPD?

A. Many therapists think that the most beneficial therapy for a child with a diagnosis of SPD is clinic-based therapy. This therapy is carried out by a therapist who specializes in sensory integration. The equipment provides an environment that is designed to give just the right challenge for your child's nervous system. The hallmark of sensory integration therapy is suspended equipment and an environment that allows for child-directed therapy. With that said, most families cannot adapt their schedules nor do they have the financial means for this kind of therapy. For these reasons, often the most effective treatment is to embed therapy throughout the day at home and in the schools.

Q. My child's therapy sessions look like play to me. What am I paying for?

A. It may not seem like therapy or "work" to you, but it's important to remember that for a child with sensory processing difficulties, playing may be the hardest thing he has to do. By making the therapy sessions fun, your child's occupational therapist is keeping him motivated so that he will continue to participate in the activities she designs for him. By utilizing fun play as a motivator, the therapist can provide your child with just the right challenge, which should encourage your child to view new sensory experiences in a positive way. This will eventually lead to him to be comfortable with or even enjoy different sensations in his world and then eventually adapt or alter how his body responds to sensory input.

If your child doesn't enjoy active play, the therapist still wants her to move. It is crucial that all children move, and children with SPD may need to be supported and encouraged to move more than the average child. You understand your body best when you have to learn to move in different and changing environments. By challenging your body to process and react to different visual, touch, proprioceptive, vestibular, and auditory information, you allow the nervous system to grow. Children with SPD require activities designed to help them move, because their nervous systems are not driven toward natural experimentation with their bodies and exploration of the world.

Q. Are mixed play groups beneficial to children with SPD?

A. Mixed play groups that involve some children with SPD and some without are great if they are set up correctly. However, if a play group has too many members with a wide variety of capabilities, this can make it less fruitful for all the children involved. If the children are all at about the same capability level and are at the point where they are actually learning from each other, this format could be a great learning experience for your child. Ask the therapy clinic or school that is sponsoring the play groups if you can observe a couple of play groups to see if you think your child would benefit from the experience.

Q. Would a mixed preschool designed for high-functioning autistic children be beneficial to a child with SPD?

A. That is a hard determination to make without knowing the school or your child's needs. But many of the strategies that are used to help children with autism learn and engage in the world around them may be very beneficial to a child with SPD. These strategies include visual schedules and visual cues for everyday activities as well as sensory strategies. Schools designed for autistic children tend to have a very structured environment, which gives a child a sense of security that allows her to work on her SPD issues.

First, go observe at the school. Then talk to the staff and find out their experience level. You can ask them a couple of questions about sensory integration to see if they have a basic understanding of SPD. Ask if they have an occupational therapist on staff or at least as a consultant. (Many autism programs are hiring OTs to consult in the classroom and help design sensory-friendly classrooms). Tell them about your child's SPD and ask the staff if they feel that the school would be a good learning environment for a child with SPD. Make sure you ask your child's occupational therapist if he or she thinks it would be a good match.

Q. What is a "brushing program"?

A. A brushing program is sometimes recommended for children who have severe tactile defensiveness. It refers to the Wilbarger Deep

Pressure and Proprioceptive Technique (DPPT), which used to be called the Wilbarger Brushing Protocol. DPPT is a specific sensory integration technique designed to help the mind and body organize and process incoming stimulation, which should lead to a decrease in defensive behavior.

The protocol requires a specific type of brush that is used to provide deep-pressure stimulation followed by gentle joint compressions. The protocol requires that the procedure be done every two hours for a certain number of days. The number of days varies depending on the child's needs and the ability of those caring for the child to administer the protocol.

A word of caution: You should not begin the Wilbarger Deep Pressure and Proprioceptive Technique on your child until an occupational therapist trained in the program has instructed you on how to administer the protocol with your child. The occupational therapist who prescribed the protocol should be monitoring its effectiveness.

Here is a brief description of the Wilbarger Deep Pressure and Proprioceptive Technique:

Brushing Step

Using a specific kind of soft, plastic surgical brush, you apply firm pressure starting at the arms, moving down toward the feet. The stomach and chest should be avoided because stimulating these areas can lead to the feeling of gagging/vomiting or urinating.

Note: Some people may be highly sensitive to this part of the protocol and may have an adverse reaction. However, within two or three administrations, the brushing part of the protocol has a calming or relaxing effect on most children. Often children will ask to be brushed when overstimulated by other types of input.

Joint Compression Step

A ten-count repetition of light pressure is applied to the joints. For example, for the elbow joint, you would place your hands on either side of the joint, close to the elbow, to stabilize it and then gently push the joint together. It is important that the joint is in alignment and that the person administering it does not use too much force.

If a child will not sit still or tolerate this, you can obtain similar deep-pressure stimulation by having the child jump on a trampoline, bounce on a ball, or do a series of exercises such as push-ups.

Oral Swipe

This last step is used for children with oral defensiveness. Often this step is not administered due to hygiene issues and safety concerns, especially when using this protocol in schools.

Q. What is Therapeutic Listening?

A. Therapeutic Listening is a listening protocol designed by Sheila Frick, an occupational therapist, that promotes the use of a sound-based intervention along with sensory integrative activities to help children with sensory difficulties. It has been documented to help children with modulation, attention, behavior, and speech and language difficulties.

In order to get your child on the Therapeutic Listening protocol, you will need to find a certified Therapeutic Listening provider. Therapists must take at least one training course to administer the protocol. Once they have completed the initial certification course, they are trained to evaluate and set up a Therapeutic Listening program for a child. They are given a certification number that allows them to order the headphones and modified CDs used in the protocol.

Following an evaluation, a therapist certified in Therapeutic Listening will set up a program that can be done at home, school, or in the community. The child is given headphones with particular acoustic specifications and a portable CD player that plays electronically engineered CDs. The headphones your child wears are unique because they allow him to hear everything around him while also listening to the modified music. Therapeutic Listening is very flexible because it is a portable program and a child does not have to be sitting still to access the benefits. As a matter of fact, it is better if your child is moving while participating in the program.

For best results, it is not recommended that your child watch TV or work on the computer while listening to the headphones, because these activities allow the brain to "check out" and the idea is to have your child's brain and body actively engaged while wearing the headphones.

Q. What is the Listening Program, and how is it different from Therapeutic Listening?

A. Both programs require special training to administer and are based on similar research. Both listening programs use electronically engineered CDs and headphones with specific acoustic specifications that make use of portable CD players. The Listening Program has a defined progression of CDs for your child to listen to, whereas the Therapeutic Listening program relies on the expertise of the therapist administering it to determine which CDs are appropriate. Both programs encourage your child to be participating in other activities while participating in the listening protocol.

The choice of programs you utilize may boil down to the program in which your therapist is certified. You should ask your child's therapist to explain what the goal is when using either program. Both programs will require your involvement.

Q. What about Auditory Integration Training?

A. Auditory Integration Training, which was developed by Guy Berard, is a more intensive program that is also more restrictive because it must be done in a clinic dedicated to Auditory Integration Training. Several occupational therapy and speech therapy clinics house these programs; visit www.aitinstitute.org for more information.

Q. Is all therapy weekly or biweekly, or are other types of therapy available?

A. Many therapists realize that not all parents have the money or the time for ongoing therapy sessions. As a result, some clinics have started doing group sessions, such as sensory-motor groups or handwriting groups. This type of therapy is usually less expensive and will last for a set number of weeks. Other occupational therapy clinics offer sensory-based play groups. Some clinics only offer them in the summer, and other clinics offer year-round groups. Call your local therapy clinic and ask what options are available.

Q. What is intensive therapy?

A. Intensive therapy, also called *treatment intensives*, requires you to make a commitment for your child to attend therapy several hours a day, every day, for one to ten weeks. It is intended for children who have very serious needs. This model will often incorporate other disciplines, such as speech therapy, behavioral therapy, music therapy, or psychology services. Many families have reported much success with intensive therapy.

This model works well for families who live in areas where regular access to treatment is not realistic or weekly sessions are not reasonable due to scheduling issues. Often, families will travel to the clinic offering treatment intensives and stay in a hotel or with friends. Some clinics have funding available to help families with the related costs.

There are intensive therapy teams throughout the country who will also come to you. This is something to consider if you live in a rural area.

Q. Are there camps devoted to working on sensory integration difficulties?

A. Yes. Camp Avanti in Wisconsin is run by some of the leading practitioners in the country and attracts a talented group of therapists every year who are dedicated to working with children with sensory processing difficulties. There are several other camps throughout the country that utilize a sensory integration approach. Make sure to call your local therapy clinics because they may be offering or sponsoring some summer-camp-type programs or be able to provide you with information about sensory camps in your area.

Camp Avanti has served children with learning disabilities since 1986 with a special sensory integration therapy program. Nearly sixty children attend this unique week-long camp each June.

Q. Are there other types of therapy besides occupational therapy?

A. A number of different therapy approaches can be taken in addition to sensory strategies. It is important when embarking on a new approach to ask specifics about the goals of the therapy and how they relate to your child's needs. Here is a list of some other therapy approaches:

- *Aquatic Therapy or Hydrotherapy*—Water-based activities that are done in warm water. Many occupational and physical therapists will conduct therapies in warm-water pools for people with neurological and orthopedic impairments. For many children with SPD, a pool can be scary; however, once they adjust to being immersed in the water, they become very secure and may even seek it out to help calm themselves. Water acts like a Lycra suit on the body, giving continuous nongraded input. Jets in a hydro spa provide increased resistance to a child's movement. Aquatic therapy programs encourage improvements in balance, bilateral control, and motor planning, as well as a general increase in body strength and body awareness.

- *Vision therapy*—Can also be referred to as eye training. A developmental optometrist will set up a program that is specific to your child's needs. The optometrist may simply recommend eye exercise or suggest that your child come in weekly for vision therapy by a vision therapist or occupational therapist who has training in this area. Note: It is imperative that you go to a developmental optometrist for this therapy. (See www.covd.org for more information.)
- *Specific nutritional diets*—In some cases, specific food allergies or intolerances of certain foods can cause behaviors that look like ADHD or SPD. If you see behaviors related to specific foods, keep records and talk to your pediatrician and a nutritionist.
- *Hippotherapy (therapeutic riding)*—Uses the sensory experience of riding a horse as well as caring for horses as a multisensory experience in a natural setting. To find a hippotherapy clinic in your area, contact www.americanhippotherapy.org.
- *Cranio-sacral/myofacial release/massage*—Some occupational therapists are trained in these therapies as well as infant massage. These therapies are considered body work and may enhance a sensory integration program. Ask your child's occupational therapist if one of these therapies would be a good complement to your child's current therapy program.

Chapter 7

YOUR CHILD AT HOME

- What advice do you have for parents of children with SPD?
- Is there a specific lifestyle change that is recommended for children with SPD?
- Is it safe to try home sensory activities I read about in a book or on the Internet?
- I was told to be very careful during swinging activities. Why?
- Are there precautions for using vestibular input at home with my child?
- My child's grandparents do not take SPD seriously. What should I tell them?
- If I home-school my child, how can I get special education services?
- The holidays are a nightmare for my child. Any ideas?
- My child with SPD has low self-esteem. How can I help?
- How do I teach my child to understand his sensory needs?
- Is there something I can do to make our mornings easier?
- My husband and I disagree on the severity of my child's sensory-seeking behavior. Who is right?
- How can I get my husband more involved in my child's therapy?
- My teenager has severe coordination difficulties but still wants to drive. How do I handle this?
- How can I help my teenager be more organized and follow through with plans?
- What is a good bedtime routine for my child with SPD?

Q. What advice do you have for parents of children with SPD?

A. The most important advice can be summarized in one word: preparation. It is vitally important to prepare your child with SPD for new experiences, as well as all experiences that your child has a history of reacting to negatively. Preparing your child means always telling him or showing him (with pictures) what is going to come next, whether it be the next hour, next day, or next week. One of the best ways to do this for younger children is to use social stories that include a picture of the child and a visual calendar. For older children, talking it through and allowing them to rehearse any situation, including social and motor type activities, is vital. Rehearse how the situation(s) may unfold and possible alternative scenarios.

Videotaping your child during different activities (such as a birthday party) and letting him watch himself in the video is a great way to prepare him for the next time he encounters that activity. However, it is crucial that you only let him watch the segments that are positive. Never allow your child to watch a video of himself behaving abnormally because that negative visual will play over and over in his head.

You, the parent, must also be prepared. Know what to expect so you can prepare your child for sensory experiences. This may mean having his favorite squeegee ball or crunchy snack available at all times, for example.

If you know your child will be encountering a highly stressful situation, make sure you have an escape plan worked out with your child that will allow him a safe refuge. This should help alleviate anxiety.

Q. Is there a specific lifestyle change that is recommended for children with SPD?

A. The number one lifestyle change that is recommended is to decrease screen time (TV and computer time) and replace it with movement-based activities. Many children with SPD prefer screen-type activities because they are more isolated and don't require brain/body communication. It is vital that your child with SPD be steered toward creative, motor-type activities. The more activities your child can do outside, the better. The nervous system must be challenged to grow through a myriad of sensory-system input in order for it to have the best chance to mature properly. I always advocate for more outside time because interaction with the natural world cannot be topped for the opportunities it provides to our nervous systems.

Q. Is it safe to try home sensory activities I read about in a book or on the Internet?

A. Any activities you choose from a book or the Internet are not necessarily going to be specific to your child's needs. So it is important to monitor your child's behavior, both physically and emotionally, during the activities. Remember, not every activity is going to be right for your child's sensory needs.

If your child indicates fear or distress during an activity, do not force the activity. See if there is a simple way to modify it to decrease his fear. The fear is based on his nervous system's reaction to the sensory input and is not under his control.

Avoid overstimulating a child by looking for cues to stop the activity, such as eye gaze aversion, pushing the activity away, uncontrollable giggling, crying, covering his eyes or ears, or tucking his head to the chest. Some children may not show overt distress. As a parent, if you can read discomfort in your child, it is time to alter or halt the activity.

Q. I was told to be very careful during swinging activities. Why?

A. Swinging activities, especially those done to alert the nervous system, have a very powerful effect on the body and brain. Some children have adverse reactions to strong vestibular input. It is important when using vestibular activities with a child who is sensory avoidant to watch for signs of overload. A child who is a sensory seeker will seek out this type of stimulation and, in a sense, "get drunk" off of it. In both cases, you want to use vestibular input in a controlled manner.

Q. Are there precautions for using vestibular input at home with my child?

A. Because vestibular input is so powerful, it is important to be very aware of signs of overstimulation. A rule of thumb when using vestibular input for children with SPD is never to force it. Their natural reactions are their nervous systems' way of communicating that they need to ease into the stimulation. During any kind of vestibular input (e.g., scooter boards, slides, swings, etc.), make sure your child is able to respond to you both visually and auditorially.

Signs of vestibular overstimulation:
- Difficulty focusing (visually) on a person or an object
- Radical/quick changes in pulse and/or respiration
- Physically listless and disoriented
- Radical changes in behavior for several minutes after ending activity, such as excessive laughing and/or hyperactivity OR unusually quiet and disengaged
- Child displays nausea, dizziness, and/or headache for several minutes after ending activity
- Physiological effects: changes in skin color (flushing, blanching) or changes in skin temperature (sweating, clamminess)

The most powerful counteractive input to overstimulation is proprioceptive input (deep pressure). If you see any of the signs listed in the previous answer, stop the vestibular stimulation and give your child deep-pressure input, such as a bear hug or have him squeeze something. Another effective tool is to have your child suck on a straw or a lemon. Ask your child to focus on something on the wall for several seconds while you help her to breathe regularly.

Note: If your child has a history of seizures, he can have strong adverse affects to rotary movement and visual stimulation. So make sure to monitor your child closely.

Q. My child's grandparents do not take SPD seriously. What should I tell them?

A. First, do not get defensive. There will be many people in your child's world, including some medical and educational professionals, who are of the same opinion as her grandparents. Regardless of their opinions, there is research to support the fact that sensory processing disorder is a real condition. You need to explain to your child's grandparents that SPD is a neurological processing difficulty. Provide them with a good resource that explains sensory processing disorder (such as this book) and ask them to learn more about it from this resource.

I recommend choosing a resource that is geared toward the nonmedical community. Here are a few:

Sensory Processing for Parents: From Roots to Wings, Judith E. Reisman

The Out-of-Sync Child Video, by Carol Kranowitz

Tools for Students, by Diana Henry

Tools for Teachers, by Diana Henry

Q. If I home-school my child, how can I get special education services?

A. Write a letter to the special education director of your school district. Even if you home-school your child, the local school is responsible for providing the extra services. Make sure you frame your letter in terms of how his "disability" is impacting his education, such as fine motor skills for writing, visual motor for copying, or behavior difficulties that interfere with learning, such as auditory and tactile sensitivities. Talk in terms of how it impacts him in the classroom setting and request an evaluation by an occupational therapist.

Note: Some charter home schools offer special education services, such as occupational therapy, speech therapy, as well as other educational services.

Q. The holidays are a nightmare for my child. Any ideas?

A. Many of us associate winter holidays with parties, presents, lots of food, and fun. But for some kids with SPD, the holidays are every sensory nightmare coming true. Visual stimulation is everywhere, and new smells, including foods, pine, and perfumes, fill the air. On top of that, kids must deal with the tactile overload of all those family members and friends kissing and hugging without invitation. Here are a few tips to help your family get through the holiday season with limited sensory meltdowns:

- Remember your child's sensory sensitivities (e.g., touch, smells, etc.).
- Steer clear of the times that malls and other places are most congested.
- Make sure family members understand that this is an unusually difficult time for your child and that hugging and kissing, even family members, is her choice.

- If you are going to holiday parties, prepare and prepare. Bring your child's favorite food. Remember that people tend to dig deep into their recipe books for holiday parties.
- If you are having a big party with lots of people attending, make sure there is a "safe" place in the house, free of people and blinking lights.
- Since routines are easily thrown aside during the holidays, make sure to discuss the changes in your child's day/week beforehand (a visual schedule may help her prepare for the changes).

It is important to keep in mind that during the holidays, sugar intake increases, bedtime routines are broken, and social demands are put upon all of us (parents and children). Mentally prepare yourself for your child to be much more sensitive, and take care not to mirror your child's frustration or add to it by becoming frustrated.

Q. My child with SPD has low self-esteem. How can I help?

A. When we consider a child's self-esteem, it helps to refer to learning disabilities expert Dr. Richard Lavoe's analogy of poker chips. We lose and gain poker chips all day long. For example, if your son gets a good grade on a test, he receives 20,000 poker chips; if he doesn't get on the soccer team, he loses 10,000; if another student makes fun of him, he loses 30,000; and at the end of the day, his bank is negative 20,000 poker chips. Children with sensory processing disorder are starting the game with fewer chips, because they continually are faced with a sensory world that is difficult to manage. It is important that the adults in your child's life be aware of this and make an effort to supply him with extra chips so that he ends each day with a positive amount in his account.

Children with sensory processing disorder tend to be more afraid to try new things than their peers because they don't always know how their bodies will react. It is very important that you help your son understand his strengths and participate in all the activities (cognitive, motor, and social) that he is good at. For instance, if he finds math challenging but will hide in his room and read for hours, work with his teachers to use his love of reading to give him more of those self-esteem poker chips. One of the best ways to do this is to encourage your child to use his strengths to help other children, either younger kids or those who aren't as strong in reading as your child. Let's face it; self-esteem poker chips that come from other kids are worth more than those coming from parents. On this same note, look for things your child can do at home and in his community that give him more chips for his self-esteem bank.

One of the keys things to remember as a parent of a child with motor difficulties is not to be the one taking away the poker chips. This means holding your tongue carefully when those clumsy moments happen.

Q. How do I teach my child to understand his sensory needs?

A. Some great tools are available to help parents, educators, and therapists teach children about their own bodies. A program that has been successful with elementary-age children is "How Does Your Engine Run?" There are also some great books to explain sensory needs to children, such as *Sensory Social Stories*. This is also a good time to share any sensory sensitivities you or a spouse may have or have had and discuss how you deal with it so your child realizes that everyone has some sensory issues. Also, talk to your child about how her sensory systems are impacting her academic, social, and movement capabilities. It is important that your child understands that she is not bad or unintelligent, but that her nervous system processes information differently and that she will need to learn to regularly use the strategies she has been taught by you and her therapist.

Q. Is there something I can do to make our mornings easier?

A. Try creating a picture schedule of the morning routine. For younger children, put a Velcro strip on laminated cardboard and attach pictures of the morning activities that your child can remove and put in an envelope as he completes each task.

Try to plan ahead as much as possible so that mornings go smoother. Choose something simple for breakfast that can be eaten on the go (e.g., peanut butter toast) if your child needs more time to get ready. Pick out your child's clothes the night before. New outfits can be tried on the night before to avoid tussling over them in the morning. To help with timing, play specific songs for specific activities. Your child will know how long each song is and will develop an internal clock for how long it takes to do various daily activities. In order to keep your child focused, you may also want to use a visual timer for specific activities such as dressing or brushing teeth.

For children who have difficulty waking up, bring them a glass of cold ice water with a straw in the mornings. This is both stimulating and hydrating. For a child who is overresponsive, start the morning off with a deep-pressure activity. This could take the form of a long, hard bear hug. (It will feel great to you, too!)

Q. My husband and I disagree on the severity of my child's sensory-seeking behavior. Who is right?

A. Differing perceptions of your child's behavior are typical because we tend to view another's actions or behavior through the lens of our own behavior. So if your husband enjoys rough-and-tumble, movement-type activities (which therapists call proprioceptive-vestibular activities), he will view your child's need for movement and deep-pressure-type activities as completely normal, which it may be. It becomes an issue when the sensory-seeking behaviors interfere with your child's ability to participate in his occupational role of being a child, such as attending school, playing with friends, or enjoying activities.

Q. How can I get my husband more involved in my child's therapy?

A. Encourage your husband to attend at least one therapy session. But, more important, realize that "dad interaction" is a gift to all children and especially to those with SPD. Dads tend to play rougher, harder, and do not tend to read as much into behaviors as moms do. They also tend to be more comfortable with allowing children to take risks. So encourage your husband to engage in as much dad-play as possible but still be aware of your son's sensory needs.

Q. My teenager has severe coordination difficulties but still wants to drive. How do I handle this?

A. If you think about how much sensory processing goes on while we drive, especially as we are learning to drive, it is amazing. Every single sensory system (except taste, one would hope) is being taxed, and it requires a great deal of motor planning. Start by breaking down the task to small, more practicable components. First, he should spend some time just sitting in a car, figuring out where to place his hands and his feet, how to move his foot from brake to accelerator and back, how to turn on the lights, and so on. Then get a road driving computer test so he can get some practice steering and turning while taking in visual input without being in a moving car. He can then try driving a golf cart or bumper cars at an amusement park or fair. When you and your son feel like he's mastered those steps, practice driving in a parking lot when no one is around. Start out by just going in a straight direction, and then practice turning and driving around obstacles.

Q. How can I help my teenager be more organized and follow through with plans?

A. Help your child identify the steps necessary to complete a task. By doing this, you are providing him with tools he can utilize independently to perform a task. When presenting directions, utilize a multi-sensory approach; use visual, auditory and gestural cues, and demonstrate the direction if possible. Help him plan out a task or a series of tasks by asking, "What materials do you need? What will be your first step?"

To aid in planning for play or projects, provide suggestions or a time for brainstorming (in the classroom with peers and at home with family members). For instance, on Friday night, plan a weekend schedule with some ideas for activities, and include steps to make it happen. The more input he receives in his home setting, the more natural it will become for him to do this on his own. Utilize a white board or chalkboard in your child's room to order the day and help keep him focused. This will also help him with projection (what will happen next). Encourage him to check off items from the white board as complete.

A "home office" provides a quiet environment to organize thoughts and focus. If possible, he should not do homework in his room, but have a predictable site that is away from the distraction of the television or other competing stimuli (except for organizing-type music). When your son does not have homework, he should still spend a set amount of time in the home office setting to pursue cognitive activities such as reading. This will make the pursuit of quieter, focused activities a routine in his day.

Q. What is a good bedtime routine for my child with SPD?

A. First, try to stay on the same sleep/wake schedule each day. A very important rule should be that the television is off for at least thirty minutes before your child's bedtime. Television is highly visually and auditorially stimulating, and most children with SPD cannot simply cut off that excitability just because you say, "Go to bed." Establish a calming bedtime routine that may consist of a warm bath and applying lotion using deep pressure (call it your child's night massage). Let your child pick out a book to bring to bed and read her a story while you are both lying on your bellies.

Keep in mind that using proprioceptive activities in a calming manner and slow rocking vestibular input should help slow your child's nervous system down. At the end of the night while your child is in bed, calmly tell her what is in store for the next day. Sometimes children become so anxious about what tomorrow will bring that they cannot fall asleep. For example, you can say, "Tomorrow you will wake up and see Mommy and Daddy, and have cereal." You can use the same approach with older children as well, but obviously you will use more appropriate language. Do not bring up things that are anxiety provoking right before your child attempts to go to sleep.

Chapter 8

SENSORY INTEGRATION STRATEGIES

- How can I help a child who is orally defensive?
- How can I help a child with tactile sensitivities who is a picky eater?
- Why does my child overstuff her mouth?
- What are some oral-motor exercises my child can do at home?
- How do I convince my child with tactile defensiveness to cut his hair?
- My four-year-old sucks his thumb constantly. How can I get him to stop?
- What strategies will help a child who is afraid of noises?
- How can I help my tactile defensive child touch different textures?
- What strategies can I use to help with my child's behavioral difficulties?
- What are some ways to help my ten-year-old with leisure and social skills?

Q. How can I help a child who is orally defensive?

A. Mix up the textures that come in contact with your child's face. Use different textured washcloths when washing his face. When drying his face, try silky cloth, coarse washcloths, and even paper towels. If your child seems reluctant, try it first on your own mouth. Make a funny face and say, "your turn." Or, let your child wipe your mouth, while you say things like "mmm that feels good!" or "that's soft." After he wipes your face, he may try to mimic your reactions and wipe his own.

When brushing your child's teeth, try using a battery-operated toothbrush. It provides stimulation without being as startling as a vibrating toothbrush. You can also use a regular toothbrush—just make sure you move all around the mouth, including brushing the tongue.

Special "NUK" brushes can be used to massage the gums. Speech therapists and occupational therapists use these brushes to help desensitize the mouth. You can also try a small finger brush that fits over the end of your finger. Once your child gets the concept of using it, you can try to get him to do it himself. Anything he can do himself will feel less invasive.

Help your child ease into different textured foods. Use some foods as vehicles for others—celery sticks to get to peanut butter, French fries to get to ketchup, chips to get to cheese dip or ranch dressing, and so on. Kids who are defensive may suck off the dip instead of taking a bite, but you can slowly encourage them to bite into it.

Make sure to offer foods of various textures for children who are orally defensive, from crackers to sliced apples to more creamy textures such as Jell-O and pudding.

Also, drinks are a great way to ease into different textures. Start with a shake that has everything smoothly blended, then slowly increase the thickness. Offer your child drinks of varying temperatures as well.

Q. How can I help a child with tactile sensitivities who is a picky eater?

A. Make sure to rule out allergies first, even with a child who has sensory defensiveness. If it is not due to allergies, picky eating may be a learned behavior. Many times, long after the sensory issue is resolved, a child continues to exhibit the learned behavior in response to the sensory issue. In that case, a behavioral approach may be the way to go.

Teri Jasman of Behavioral Intervention Associates suggests the following step-by-step approach for picky eaters. Once your child tolerates a step, move on to the next step.

- Select a food that is similar to one of the foods your child already eats, such as a different shaped pasta noodle or a different flavored cracker.
- During snack time or meal time, place a small amount of the new food on a separate plate next to your child's plate. Teri suggests bringing your child's attention to the new food by eating some and commenting on how yummy it tastes.
- Once he tolerates the new food, put it on his plate. He doesn't have to eat it, but just be comfortable with the new food being on his plate.
- Now model touching the food and have your child do the same. Make sure you establish a set number of times your son needs to touch the food so it is clear. For example, "we're going to touch it two times."
- The next step is to have the child touch the food. To make this more concrete, you can have a food such as crackers on one plate and have the child move them to another plate.
- Now have your son touch the food to his lips. Teri suggests saying, "give the food a kiss three times."

- Now the food goes on the tongue.
- Next, place one or two bites on a plate and have the child place the food on his tongue and eat the bites of food. Over time, you can increase the amount of food.

Every child will integrate a new food at a different rate. Your son may run through these steps in a week or it may take months depending on his sensitivities, the foods you use, and how systematic you are in introducing a new food.

Q. Why does my child overstuff her mouth?

A. Special note: Children who are adopted from orphanages may display "overstuffing" behaviors, which may have a sensory as well as a survival component. See Chapter 15 for recommendations on overstuffing for internationally adopted children.

Many children who have low muscle tone will "overstuff" their mouths because they don't have good oral sensory awareness and most likely lack good oral-motor control. By stuffing their mouths with food, they are increasing the sensory input to the sensory and motor nerve fibers in their mouths and surrounding jaw. This gives them more information about where their tongue is, how wide the jaw is open, and may make it easier to chew. Ask either an occupational therapist or a speech therapist to give you an oral-motor diet for your daughter as well as some "oral-motor work." Both occupational therapy and speech therapy can address oral-motor issues.

You want to start getting things in your child's mouth that provide input. Although it's candy, taffy gives off a lot of proprioceptive input. Steak cut into strips allows your child to hold one side and literally gnaw on the other side. This is a good way to provide oral input and get a little protein at the same time (use sirloin steak, it is the toughest). Apples provide a lot of crunch and feedback, and frozen fruit helps wake up the mouth. Sucking something thick through a straw at the beginning of the meal will also provide some proprioceptive input. Some therapists use Pop Rocks candy or any kind of fizzy candy to engage the fine muscles of the mouth; the tongue gets a workout just trying to figure out where the explosion is coming from.

Q. What are some oral-motor exercises my child can do at home?

A.

- Give your child some chew tube, available online from places like therapro.com.
- Bubbles everywhere! Bubbles are a great motivator for getting those lips together and blowing. There are so many different shapes of wands that you can mix it up and surprise your child with new bubbles to keep her interest. If your daughter has difficulties, first demonstrate for her and then let her practice in front of a mirror. She can practice in the bathtub or outside to avoid sticky bubble residue on your floor.
- Sucking liquid through different types of straws is a great game.
- Have cotton ball races on the kitchen counter by using a straw to blow the cotton ball across the table.
- Put peanut butter on the roof of your child's mouth and get her to lick it off. Also, use sticky candy liquid on her lips and get her to lick it off. Both of these will help her with tongue control and knowing where her tongue is in her mouth.
- You can teach your daughter "the nose controls the tongue" game.

Push on nose—tongue sticks out, push nose to one side—tongue moves to that side, push nose up—tongue tries to reach nose, push on nose again—tongue moves back into mouth.

Q. How do I convince my child with tactile defensiveness to cut his hair?

A.

- Role play getting haircuts. Let your child pretend to cut your hair, using his hands as scissors. Then pretend to cut his hair.
- You can create a sensory social story about going to the barber or you can look into buying a social story that is already written. Go to Carol Cray's web page for more information (www.thegraycenter.org). Also check out www.sandbox-learning.com, a website that allows you to create your own social stories.
- Bring your child along when you or your spouse gets a haircut.
- Before he gets his haircut, visit the barber and make sure she understands your child's sensory needs.
- Provide your own cape made from a towel and a safety pin.
- Make sure that he wears a button-up shirt that can be taken off and shaken to get the hair off, or bring an extra shirt that he can change into.
- Right before he is going to get his hair cut, give him a head and neck massage or use a vibrating hairbrush to give extra deep-pressure input before the light touch of the haircut.
- Make sure you and your child decide on a haircut reward before the haircut. (He can even take a picture of it with him to look at while getting the haircut).

Q. My four-year-old year sucks his thumb constantly. How can I get him to stop?

A. If you are looking at your son through a sensory processing lens, this is an adaptive sensory-calming activity. Firm oral stimulation is extremely calming due to the rhythmic proprioceptive input that it supplies to the oral/facial area. The key is to teach your child that his thumb is for bedtime and naptime first, and then try to replace the thumb sucking during the day with other oral-stimulation activities.

Q. What strategies will help a child who is afraid of noises?

A. The following activity can help increase your child's ability to discriminate different sounds and desensitize him to "scary noises." You or your child's therapist can tape record different noises (such as emergency sirens, a vacuum cleaner, a toilet flushing, bells, etc.) and then make matching pictures for each noise (pictures of a fire truck, a vacuum cleaner, etc.). The noises should be taped with about ten seconds between them, and during each noise, your child holds up the picture of the corresponding noise.

Then, when your child hears the same noise during the normal course of the day, you or the teacher can say, "that's the lunch bell" and hold up the corresponding picture. This decreases a child's fear of the unexpected noise.

Here are more auditory strategies to try with your child:

- Depending on your child's needs, use the appropriate type of music. For calming sounds, use soft music such as Mozart. For alerting sounds, use music with a driving beat, such as rock.
- Earmuffs and headphones are great for blocking out noises your child dislikes (such as the garbage truck). However, it is important to note that these are just a band-aid; you must still address the underlying processing problems.
- Create an auditorially pleasing environment in your child's room with white noise, trickling water, and soft background music.
- It is important to keep in mind that children with auditory sensitivities can be defensive to high-pitched voices.

- Anytime you can link music and movement together it helps promote vestibular-auditory information.
- Ask your child's occupational therapist about different listening programs, such as Therapeutic Listening or the Listening Program.

Q. How can I help my tactile defensive child touch different textures?

A. When a child is tactilely defensive, a combination of bottom up strategies (sensory integration therapy/strategies) with top down strategies (behavioral/learning strategies) seems to be most effective for helping a child engage in her world through touch. For example, if your child resists touching anything messy: first suggest that she watch as you play with shaving cream and then reward her with something tangible (a food item or play toy that motivates them) for watching. Once she is comfortable with watching, encourage your child to help clean up the shaving cream with a big sponge, again rewarding her with something tangible. Once she is successful with this, see if you can get her to touch the shaving cream with her fingertips (if you can evoke the help of siblings, this may be more motivating for your child), then again reward her. Continue this until she has become comfortable with different textures, then gradually decrease the rewards over time. Combining behavorial and sensory strategies is a very effective way of easing a child through defensiveness in other sensory items as well.

Q. What strategies can I use to help with my child's behavioral difficulties?

A. The key thing to remember with sensory-based behaviors is that trying to eliminate the behavior without a substitute way for your child to meet the sensory need may lead to an even worse behavior. Here are some tips to keep in mind when addressing sensory-based behaviors:

- Sensory diets can be extremely effective (see Chapter 6).
- Regular sensory-based activities such as jumping on a trampoline or bouncy ball, playing hoppity-hop through the house, eating crunchy foods, or listening to rhythmic music are essential.
- Consider altering your child's regular environment (his room, playroom, etc.) to match it to his stimulation level.
- Teach your child how to quickly and effectively communicate his sensory fears in any situation.
- Remember to reward the flip side (positive behaviors).

Q. What are some ways to help my ten-year-old with leisure and social skills?

A. Consider getting your child started on long-term planning projects, such as building train tracks and a model town. This activity would require a long-term commitment as well as planning and continued attention from your child. Other ideas in this vein are model cars and airplanes. You could even build a small clubhouse in your backyard with help from friends and parents. Start with a building plan, a checklist of needed materials, and projected timeline.

Also consider theater or pantomime classes at a local theater. Games like Pictionary, charades, and Taboo all require planning and reasoning, as well as interacting with others. Increase motor-type structured and unstructured activities, such as hiking, swimming, and playing outdoor games with friends. You may need to help your child structure the background for activities and give her hints on things she can do.

Chapter 9

SCHOOL-BASED THERAPY

- My child is struggling at school. How do I get help?
- Are the eligibility criteria for school-based OT the same at every school?
- What areas of need can the school occupational therapist work on?
- What if my child's school district does not endorse Sensory Processing Disorder as a reason for therapy?
- What should I expect from the school occupational therapy services?
- What if my child's school occupational therapist isn't doing enough to help my child?
- What are the different types of school-based occupational therapy?
- Can my child get speech therapy at school?
- My eighteen-month-old may need therapy. Will the schools help me?
- What is IDEA?
- What is Response to Intervention (RTI)?
- What is an IEP?
- What is a 504 plan?
- What is a behavior plan?
- Will my child's school understand that his behavior is due to sensory processing difficulties?

Q. My child is struggling at school. How do I get help?

A. Contact the school and ask how to have your child evaluated under the Individuals with Disabilities Education Act (IDEA). Under this act and other mandates, your child may qualify for school-based occupational therapy.

To be eligible for school-based OT service, students must:

- Be identified as having a disability that interferes with education
- Have sensorimotor problems that interfere with their ability to manage classroom materials or their self-care needs in school
- Need OT intervention to become more independent or better able to participate in school activities

Before your child can be evaluated at school, you must be notified with a description of any evaluation that the school plans to perform. You must sign a consent form giving your approval before evaluations can proceed.

The professionals evaluating your child will review his files, talk to his teachers and you, and, depending on the type of evaluation, most likely observe your child in his role as a student.

Then a multidisciplinary team will conduct further evaluations according to your child's educational needs, and each professional will write a report based on the findings. You can request to receive a copy of the report before meeting with the team to discuss the results. If something isn't clear in the report, you should ask questions until you have a complete understanding of the content.

Once all team members have finished their evaluations, there will be a meeting at which the parents are present to discuss the results of the evaluations. Based on the results of the various evaluations and input from all parties, including you, the parent, an individual education plan (IEP) will be discussed and, if agreed upon, put in place.

Q. Are the eligibility criteria for school-based OT the same at every school?

A. Although the criteria should be the same, some schools interpret the criteria differently, which allows the evaluating therapist more leeway to address each child's needs. However, because of a new mandate known as Response to Intervention (RTI), many schools are revising their approaches to OT service. Some schools may recommend that the occupational therapist observe and screen a student and then develop a plan on ways to provide in-class strategies that help a student maximize her potential in the classroom. This approach can be very effective in catching students before they need special education services. It allows the therapist to intervene before sensory processing difficulties result in behavioral, social, or academic problems.

Q. What areas of need can the school occupational therapist work on?

A. Your child's school occupational therapist may work on any of the following areas if they are impeding your child's ability to access the educational curriculum.

- Fine and gross motor skills
- Visual motor skills and visual processing skills
- Sensory processing skills as they relate to educational performance, including academics, behavior, and socialization
- Activities of daily living, such as feeding, dressing, and hygiene
- Positioning and functional mobility
- Assistive technology and adaptive devices

Q. What if my child's school district does not endorse Sensory Processing Disorder as a reason for therapy?

A. Steer clear of the words *sensory integration* and talk in terms of "skill deficits." Make sure the goals you are approving for your child promote or improve learning and behavior within the academic setting. For example, if your child is highly distracted by visual or auditory information, which impacts her ability to attend class, the goal may be written: "Given a verbal prompt, Susie will attend to a writing task for ten minutes without additional prompting with 100 percent accuracy in three out of four trials as observed by teacher and therapist." Although your daughter's distraction in school is due to a sensory issue, the goal does not incorporate sensory-type wording. It is written in such a way that the OT can work with both the teacher and your child on visual and auditory strategies, and make classroom modifications to reach a goal of increased attention.

Q. What should I expect from the school occupational therapy services?

A. The following is a list of some of the services the school occupational therapist can provide. But keep in mind that most OTs in school settings are stretched thin. You may want to begin with a certain number of direct services and then move to a consult model that is designed to support the classroom teacher as well as your child in the classroom environment.

Indirect services the OT could provide:

- Explanations to the other school professionals working with your child concerning how his medical and/or sensorimotor difficulties impact his role as a student
- Adaptations for your child's access to the physical environment

- Suggestions for modifications to promote increased independence during academic work
- Consultation with your child's PE teacher to make him aware of your child's sensorimotor issues (this consultation is very important)

Direct services the OT could provide:

- All of the above services
- Consultation on specific sensory strategies that may be impacting your child's behavior as well as attention and task management skills
- A sensory diet or a sensory program designed specifically to help your child gear himself for his role as a student (from social interaction to sitting at a desk for long periods)
- Direct help with self-help skills such as toileting and feeding
- Design and implementation of fine motor and visual motor programs that promote and enhance fine motor skills
- Suggestions for activities that can be carried out at home that promote sensory organization as well as focus on particular skill development

Q. What if my child's school occupational therapist isn't doing enough to help my child?

A. Set up a time to talk to your child's occupational therapist to discuss your concerns. If you cannot get a meeting set up in a timely manner, ask the school personnel for the OT's school email address. Contact the OT with your concerns and ask if he or she would be able to assist your child in those areas. Most school-based occupational therapists have large caseloads and often wish they could spend more time with each child. They are usually extremely busy and may not be aware of specific concerns. Set up a meeting or send an email directly to the OT so that he or she will be aware of your concerns.

Q. What are the different types of school-based occupational therapy?

A. There are three primary types of service delivery models in the schools: direct, consultation, and monitoring. Direct therapy has several purposes. It is used when direct intervention is needed to teach a student a new skill, and also as a way of gathering more information about a student for ongoing consultation. The information gathered from direct therapy allows the OT to see how effective a program will be for a student before teaching it to caregivers.

Consultation is a process that helps teachers and parents alter how they view their child's performance or behavior. Through a mutual partnership, the therapist provides the tools and education the parents and teachers need to help the child on an ongoing basis. When working with older children, the therapist's goal is to involve the child in the learning process, with the child ultimately being responsible for implementing what she has learned in therapy. Occupational therapists consult directly with educators as well as students to help them become more effective at helping a particular student and/or the whole class. Consultation may be the most effective service delivery model, as it has a more sustained impact on both students and educators. It is important to understand that effective consultation requires much time and work by the occupational therapist because she must understand the role of the student and the teacher and help both be more effective in those roles.

Monitoring is an indirect service. The occupational therapist teaches certain skills to a teacher or parent such as positioning, use of adaptive equipment, or how to implement   specific handwriting program. The occupational therapist is responsible for monitoring the implementation and effectiveness of the program.

Q. Can my child get speech therapy at school?

A. The procedure for obtaining speech therapy is generally similar to obtaining other special education services. The key difference is that unlike occupational and physical therapy, speech therapy is a stand-alone service. So if your child qualifies as speech and language impaired, she can receive direct/consult speech services in school without having any other special education services. Share your concerns with the school and request that your child be evaluated by the school speech pathologist. Keep in mind that school-based speech services have strict qualifying criteria.

Q. My eighteen-month-old may need therapy. Will the schools help me?

A. Because your child is not yet three years old, you will need to contact the state health department or education department to see if they offer an early intervention program. Through this program, you can have your child evaluated and, if he qualifies, receive services free of charge. Your child's pediatrician or your local school district should have the contact information for the early intervention agency in your area. If you are having difficulty getting information from those sources, call the National Dissemination Center for Children with Disabilities (800) 695–0285 and it will provide you with the contact information for early intervention for your state. The state office will be able to tell you which agency services your area. Note that if the waiting list is long, you may want to go to a private clinic. Also, some clinics contract with the state to provide services free of charge.

Q. What is IDEA?

A. IDEA stands for the Individual with Disabilities Education Act. It is a national law first enacted in 1975 (reauthorized and updated in 2004) that ensures children with disabilities have access to a fair and appropriate education. IDEA details how states and public agencies provide early intervention, special education, and related services to children.

IDEA defines children with disabilities as being between the ages of three and twenty-two and having one or more of the following conditions:

- Mental retardation
- Speech and language impairment
- Visual impairment (including blindness)
- Hearing impairment
- Emotional disturbance
- Orthopedic impairment
- Traumatic brain injury
- ADHD/ADD
- Other health impairments
- Autism
- Specific learning disabilities (this is often how children with visual/motor/handwriting difficulties qualify)

You can find more detailed information at the government website http://idea.ed.gov.

Q. What is Response to Intervention (RTI)?

A. Response to Intervention (RTI) was created when Congress reauthorized and revamped IDEA to state that schools will "not be required to take into consideration whether a child has a severe discrepancy between achievement and intellectual ability." RTI provides academic intervention at the beginning stages of noticed academic struggles, and was developed by researchers as an alternative approach to the discrepancy model. It mandates that schools intervene early in attempt to avert academic failure. It requires frequent measurement of progress, as well as more research-based instructional interventions for children who continue to struggle in the academic setting.

Q. What is an IEP?

A. An individualized education plan (IEP) details the special education and related services that the child is to receive, based on input from the educational team, the parents, and the child, when appropriate. It is a legal, written, binding document that is based upon the evaluations of the school professionals, as well as other special consultants and, when necessary, the parents and the child. The IEP is created at a meeting between the school professionals and parents, which is set at a mutually agreeable time.

It is important to remember that you are an equal partner (by law) in the IEP process, meaning that no part of the IEP can be carried out without your approval. The school district and you must agree to sign the IEP before special education services can begin, and if at any time your child's services will change, a new IEP meeting must be held, accompanied by a written IEP. Based on new rules for IEP meetings, the IEP meeting can be held with your approval via phone conference call or video conference, or you can give approval to the school to make changes without holding a new IEP meeting. Once the initial IEP has taken place, there will be annual IEP meetings held to review your child's progress and plan goals for the following year. If at any time, you are concerned about your child's progress or feel that there should be a change in your child's educational plan, you can request an IEP meeting. Remember that the IEP is a legal, binding document.

It is important to be well prepared for your child's IEP meeting. Review all of your child's evaluations and assessments. Create a folder that contains all of this information, including school assessments, outside assessments, as well as any pertinent medical information, especially medications. Some parents choose to keep small amounts of sample schoolwork in their child's folder. This is especially important if you are moving to a new school.

Share any assessments from outside agencies with the director of special education. Based on the assessments and your observations, write down your concerns and educational goals for your child. For example, "I want to see my son write a sentence, or pay attention during math, or make friends." Make sure you also write down your child's strengths. This will help the team capitalize on high-interest areas for your child.

Before the meeting, try to talk to some of the therapists and teachers that are on the IEP team. This will give you better insight into what the professionals are thinking about for your child. If there are placement considerations for your child, visit the classrooms or schools being offered as options so that you are clear in the meeting when professionals start talking about program options.

Remember that you are a crucial part of the IEP team and that your wishes for your child need to be heard by the IEP team. If you think you may need some support at the meeting, bring a friend, family member, or an advocate who can take notes for you and help you remember the points you wanted to make at the meeting.

Q. What is a 504 plan?

A."504" refers to Section 504 of the Federal Rehabilitation Act (1973), which is separate from IDEA. It requires all agencies that receive federal monies to provide access to individuals with disabilities. In the school setting, if a child does not qualify under IDEA, she may be deemed eligible for services under Section 504. The school will evaluate eligibility based on:

- Whether the child has a physical/medical impairment
- Whether this impairment hinders the child's access to the physical/educational environment
- Whether this impairment hinders the child's learning
- The types of accommodations the child requires to receive a public education

Q. What is a behavior plan?

A. It is a plan designed to teach your child replacement behaviors rather than using punishment strategies. The plan can be created by a behaviorist, therapist, school psychologist, or your child's teacher. The best plans come from a team effort and include input from you (the parent). More and more schools are using a behavior plan designed by the consultant Diana Browning Wright, called a "Behavior Support Plan." No matter who creates the plan, it must be reviewed and approved by the parent(s).

These are the steps that should be involved in creating a Positive Behavior Support Plan:

- First define the behavior in observable, measurable terms without judgment. For example, instead of saying, "he throws a fit before lunch," say, "he pounds the desk and yells when the lunch bell rings."
- Then decide which behaviors are impeding your child's learning or the learning of others.

- Then gather information. A formal assessment may be used to obtain more in-depth information and shed light on other behaviors as well as motivators.
- Record what happened just prior to the behavior, what time of day it happened, and who was present.
- Note the consequence of the child's behaviors. This may include natural consequences as well as those imposed by school staff or parents. This does not necessarily mean punishment; it could mean other children move away from him, or he has limited time to eat lunch because he spends some of the time being coaxed to lunch. Sometimes the consequence is additional attention from a teacher or parent.

A Positive Behavior Support Plan first attempts to understand *why* the behavior is occurring by locating the need that the behavior is meeting for the child. For example, the child who gets up in the middle of the class and runs around the room may be trying to meet a sensory need and organize himself. The second part of the behavior plan identifies how the environment can be altered to help reduce the student's need to use that behavior. For example, the teacher could move the student to the front row so that he is no longer distracted by others. The third part of the plan is made up of strategies that educators and other team members can use to support the student. These strategies use identified positive replacement behaviors that can help the child meet his sensory needs.

Q. Will my child's school understand that his behavior is due to sensory processing difficulties?

A. Many educators understand that behavioral issues are often linked to sensory processing issues. Below you will find a simple flowchart that can be used to help your child's teacher and other team members brainstorm possible causes of observable behaviors and find appropriate replacement behaviors (or behavior strategies) that can be taught.

You can download a useable version of this chart at www.babystepstherapy.com.

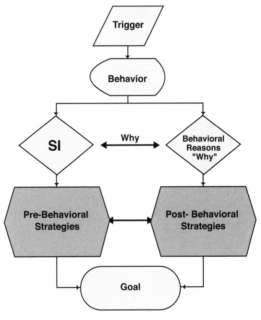

Delaney & Delaney 2006

Trigger—The event that may have prompted the behavior, such as a change in schedule or a new person entering a room.

Behavior—The observable description of the reaction/action.

Behavioral reasons "why"—Avoidance of a nonpreferred task, perceived social embarrassment, etc.

SI (sensory integration) reasons "why"—Noise overload, fear of touch, visual overload, etc.

Pre-behavioral strategies—Activities such as sensory diets or environmental sensory modifications.

Post-behavioral strategies—Strategies for after a behavior has occurred, such as calming time, removal from the situation, verbal cueing to return to work, etc.

Goal—the desired outcome of parent, staff, or child—for example, that the child will transition to lunch without incident.

Chapter 10

STRATEGIES FOR SCHOOL SUCCESS

- When my child gets overwhelmed, he hits other people, and this is causing problems at school. What should I do?
- My eight-year-old child struggles with handwriting. What can I do to help her?
- Why does my child keep breaking his pencil at school?
- My child starts school soon. How do I prepare her teacher?
- How do I make sure the teacher understands and follows through on our conversation?
- What if my child's teacher is not making the accommodations we discussed?
- How do I prepare my sensory-sensitive child for the first day of school?
- When I pick my child up from school, he has a meltdown. Why?
- How can I help my child decompress from the school day?
- How can I help my child better handle the school lunchroom?
- I don't care if my child is "cool," I just don't want him to be ostracized. How can I help?
- How can I meet other parents of children with SPD in my child's school?
- What advice can I give my child's kindergarten teacher to prepare the classroom for my sensory-seeking child?
- What advice can I give my child's kindergarten teacher to prepare the classroom for my sensory-avoidant child?

Q. When my child gets overwhelmed, he hits other people, and this is causing problems at school. What should I do?

A. Your child needs to be on a sensory diet. If he is not getting occupational therapy in the school, request that an OT consult with the teacher on his sensory issues. Spend some time observing him in the classroom (preferably where he cannot see you) so you can play "sensory detective." Try to narrow down what is triggering his hitting behavior. Also try a sensory behavior story like the one shown below. Use the words given for each page and put your child's picture with the corresponding action on that page.

Page 1: "Kind hands stay in my lap." (picture of your child with hands in lap)

Page 2: "Kind hands hold hands gently." (picture of your child holding hands gently)

Page 3: "Kind hands give friends high fives." (picture of your child giving a high five)

Page 4: "When I have kind hands, friends smile and stand next to me." (picture of your child standing next to a friend)

Page 5: "When my hands are not kind, friends cry and get mad. Friends do not play with me when my hands are not kind" (picture of an unhappy friend)

Page 6: "Sometimes I get frustrated. Then I will use my hands to squeeze toys." (picture of your son with a sensory squeeze toy)

Page 7: "I will try to remember to have kind hands so friends will smile and play with me." (picture of your son playing with friends)

Q. My eight-year-old child struggles with handwriting. What can I do to help her?

A. Handwriting is another one of the wonderfully complex skills we take for granted. When a child continues to have difficulty with handwriting, it is important to have the underlying processing skills examined (visual skills, visual processing/visual motor, and motor planning skills). Remember, vestibular, proprioceptive, and tactile skills lay the foundation for more complex motor planning skills, such as handwriting.

First, make sure your child is using proper posture during handwriting. To help improve her positioning, she can practice writing on a vertical surface, which puts the wrist in a naturally good position and works on shoulder and arm strengthening. Fine motor games (see Chapter 16 for activities) promote hand and finger strengthening. Have your child practice writing letters with her eyes closed so she can develop a kinesthetic feel for how letters are formed. To work on visual processing skills, encourage activities such as word finding games, mazes, and *Where's Waldo?* books. Outdoor ball activities also promote visual skills.

You can also make modifications to the various tools your child uses for handwriting.

Consider using raised line paper, which gives tactile information about where each line is and makes it easier to keep letters on the lines when writing. She can also use a blank piece of paper below the line she is writing on to help her keep her place. Also take into account ergonomic issues, such as desk and chair height, and adjust them accordingly.

Consider buying a plastic spacer that can take the place of the child using her own hand as a spacer when writing. It is shaped like a hand with a pointer index finger, and can help your child not scrunch the letters together. You can also try a product called a space stick. You can obtain these through therapy websites, a teacher supply store, or at www.superduper.com. Or you can teach your child to use the index finger of the opposite hand as a spacer between words. She can also try different pencil grips and adjust her hand weight to increase her proprioceptive input.

Q. Why does my child keep breaking his pencil at school?

A. Your child probably does not register the amount of pressure he is putting on the pencil. Or, it could be a strategy so he can get up and sharpen his pencil because he needs to move around. If he says he isn't doing it on purpose, then he is probably not registering how much pressure he is putting on the pencil. Explain to the teacher that your child's proprioceptive and tactile senses are not providing him with enough input for him to grade his pressure. In addition to sensory activities, there are also strategies you and your child's teacher can use to help him understand how much pressure he is using when writing. Have him write on a piece of paper that is on Styrofoam. That way, when he pushes too hard, his pencil sinks into the Styrofoam, giving him feedback that he is pressing too hard. Plus, his pencil won't break!

Q. My child starts school soon. How do I prepare her teacher?

A. First, make it clear to the school principal that you need to know who your daughter's teacher will be before school starts, so that you can meet with him or her about your child's specific needs. Make sure you schedule time to talk to your child's teacher before that first day of school. This will help defer any possible assumptions that the teacher may make about your child's behavior and intellect. For example, if your child is likely to react negatively to the school bell or needs extra time and physical prompting to follow directions, tell her teacher.

Choose a time to meet with your child's teacher other than the standard open house night, and make sure you communicate that this meeting is to help the teacher as much as to help your child. Approach the meeting with the assumption that the teacher wants to help your child, as most people did not become teachers for the money, but rather because they want to help children succeed. The teacher may appear confused or apprehensive, but do your best not to become defensive. Remember that your child's teacher is part of a team of people that you need to help your child. Write down some of your major concerns and go over them with the teacher. If your child has been receiving therapy, share the strategies you have been given by the occupational therapist.

Make it clear that you are available to answer any questions she may have about your child. Ask your child's occupational therapist if it is okay to give her phone number and/or email address to the teacher. Finally, ask if you can schedule a time other than open house to visit the classroom with your child. Let your child's teacher know that you don't want to take up a lot of time (ten minutes or so).

Q. How do I make sure the teacher understands and follows through on our conversation?

A. The teacher's reception of the information you give her and the adjustments she makes to help your child in the classroom will depend on several variables. These include the number of kids in her class, her past experience educating different types of learners, her personality, her training, as well as her own personal experience as a parent or caregiver. So talking to your child's teacher does not guarantee anything, but you will be able to tell a lot about the teacher by meeting with her. Also, giving the teacher the impression that you want to work together and make those first few weeks as enjoyable as possible for everyone will likely gain you an ally. You will also have gone a long way to decreasing the possibility of your child's sensory reactions being seen by her teacher as misbehavior or evidence of cognitive limitations.

Q. What if my child's teacher is not making the accommodations we discussed?

A. If your child's difficulties impact her ability to access the curriculum, she may qualify for an individualized education plan (IEP). Your child can be evaluated by a school-based occupational therapist who will then suggest these accommodations as part of the child's IEP. Because an IEP is a legally binding document, the teacher will have to follow the recommendations therein and make the appropriate accommodations for your child. If your child does not qualify for special education services or does not currently have an IEP in place, talk to the principal and see if you can have the school's occupational therapist consult with your child's teacher.

Q. How do I prepare my sensory-sensitive child for the first day of school?

A. Ask if your child can tour the classroom sometime when there isn't a mob of kids there. During your visit, take pictures of the classroom, your child in the classroom, and your child's teacher standing with your child. Make sure you take pictures of the lunchroom, the principal (if possible), as well as any special assembly rooms.

Now, with those pictures, create a simple "picture book" about your child's new school. Each page should have one big picture and a few simple words. If you don't have personalized photos of every situation, download a picture from the Internet. Below is an example book:

"I'm going to school." (picture of your child smiling)

"This is my new school." (picture of school building)

"This is my new teacher." (picture of teacher)

"This is my classroom." (picture of classroom)

"At school we sit at desks." (picture of desks)

"And we sit in a circle." (picture of students sitting in a circle)

"At school I will learn to write and read." (pictures of books)

"I will meet new friends." (download picture of a group of kids from the Internet)

"There will be new noises at school." (picture of a bell)

"Going to school makes me happy." (picture of your child smiling)

Q. When I pick my child up from school, he has a meltdown. Why?

A. School is a very demanding place for children with sensory processing disorder. They are required to be still for long periods of time, respond to auditory and visual information quickly, and then take in and respond to all the social cues around them. Your child is probably working very hard to "hold it together" during school and simply unravels when he is with someone safe (and who is safer than a parent?).

Q. How can I help my child decompress from the school day?

A. First, talk to your child about the fact that she needs some down-time after a long day at school. Explain to her that most adults also require "regrouping" time after a long day at work. Then make a list together of some possible things that comfort or calm her that she can look forward to right after school. For instance, place Therapeutic Listening or Listening Program headphones in the car for when you pick her up from school, and include a selection of prescribed calming music targeted toward centering and transitions (try one of Vital Links' "Gear Shifter" CDs). For more information about Therapeutic Listening, see Chapter 6. Also try to have a fruit smoothie or other thick drink ready for her to drink through a straw when she gets in the car.

Allow your child to look at a photo album in the car of her doing activities that she does at home or for fun. This can help her visualize doing activities that she perceives as fun or relaxing, which will aid her in the transition from a more taxing environment. If possible, do not schedule another activity directly after school, since your child needs time to regulate herself. Consider asking the teacher to arrange a short "break time" for your child during the school day, so that she can do some of her sensory-regulation activities.

Q. How can I help my child better handle the school lunchroom?

A. School lunchrooms give many of us headaches, so just imagine what the impact is on a child with sensory processing disorder. If the lunchroom is overwhelming, see if your child and a few other kids can eat in a quieter place together. This is also a great way to work on social skills in a small-group setting. Many schools are now promoting "lunch clubs" for students who need a quieter setting for lunch. But if your child wants to be in the big lunchroom with all her friends, ask her what she doesn't like about it. If it is the noise, she can wear headphones with low music or no music. Some kids have difficulty with things like carrying their lunch tray; if that is the case, you can work on it at home (practice carrying a tray with different things on it) or consider having your child bring her lunch to school. Most important, acknowledge that the lunchroom is an overwhelming environment and help your child think of ways she can regulate herself. This sets the stage for her to regulate herself in different environments throughout her life.

Q. I don't care if my child is "cool," I just don't want him to be ostracized. How can I help?

A. Understanding how your child's sensory system impacts his ability to move in and out of social situations is key. First, discuss social situations with your child and tell him that many children, as well as adults, feel uncomfortable around others. Help him with the language to describe how he is feeling, such as, "I am afraid someone is going to bump into me so I stay away from people because I don't like that kind of touch." Once he is able to understand why certain social situations make him feel uncomfortable, then you will both be better able to find sensory and social strategies that make him feel more empowered. Next, talk to your child's teacher and see if there are one or two children that he seems to play well with or who appear to be more accepting of his sensory behaviors. Once you find out this information, cultivate these relationships by calling their parents and explain to them some of your child's fears. Then set up buddy time. The good thing is that you can help structure some of this interaction so that both children have fun. Also, ask your child's occupational therapist to work on some strategies that he can use so that other kids may see him as fun and join in.

Q. How can I meet other parents of children with SPD in my child's school?

A. Ask the school OT if you can help organize an in-service that she conducts to address sensory issues that school-aged children may face. If you are going to ask her to put this together, be willing to help organize it, as well as get the word out to other parents. You can also organize a support group to meet at school. Ask the school if they can have students bring the invitation home to their parents. In order to meet other parents who may not be associated with the school, look for the parent network on the SPD Network website: www.spdnetwork.org. This network is an excellent place to start if you have challenges finding assistance at the school.

Q. What advice can I give my child's kindergarten teacher to prepare the classroom for my sensory-seeking child?

A. Most children who are sensory seeking are all over the place, especially in a new environment. They have difficulty focusing and move from one thing to another quickly. A lot of sensory seekers are "touchers" and feel the need to touch everything they see, sometimes more than once. This is the child who teachers may see as ADHD or purposefully acting up, or rough with other children. This child will be told, "keep your hands to yourself," "sit still," and "listen" many times until he learns how to control his sensory-seeking body.

Makes sure the teacher knows that your child needs structure. He will require a lot of outside cues, direction from the teacher, and pictures of how to control his body, so that he doesn't hurt himself or others. Pictures of what to do with his hands and what *not* to do with his hands, will help guide him in the new classroom environment. He may have to be told, "This is how we touch others' bodies," while the teacher/parent models gentle touch. Equally as important as structure are scheduled movement breaks, which allow him to move his body and feel free to explore his environment.

Q. What advice can I give my child's kindergarten teacher to prepare the classroom for my sensory-avoidant child?

A. The child who is sensory avoidant is going to react by withdrawing or fleeing when sensory information is overwhelming. Such children often interpret everyday stimulation as noxious stimulation and respond accordingly.

The environment for a sensory-avoidant child should have minimal "surprise" sensory input. The environment should be sensory soothing. There should also be plenty of preparation for change, such as pictures or soothing auditory input to indicate that it is time to transition to a new activity or place. The teacher should understand that this child may withdraw or react negatively to a new person or activity, and be reassured that it is important not to rush or push her into new situations without adequate support.

Chapter 11

SOCIAL SITUATIONS

- How can I get my sensory-sensitive child ready for a family trip to Disneyland?
- What can I do to help my child sit through a church service?
- Are there any alternatives to play groups?
- How should I prepare my child for a Fourth of July party?
- How do I plan a birthday party for my teenager who is easily overstimulated?
- What are some tips for helping my teenager in social situations, especially parties or large gatherings?
- Should I enroll my child in a social skills training group?
- How do I stop my child from throwing temper tantrums in public?
- How can we make going to a restaurant less of an ordeal?
- How can I help my child enjoy her friends' birthday parties?
- My child "freaks" at the thought of going to the dentist. What can I do?
- My child's grandparents give her gifts that she really likes, but her facial expression is either blank or pained. Her grandparents think she doesn't like the gifts. Is there anything I can do?

Q. How can I get my sensory-sensitive child ready for a family trip to Disneyland?

A. A child with sensory processing difficulties is going to need a lot of "stimulation protection" so that the trip isn't traumatic for him and the whole family. Here are some pre-trip recommendations:

- Try to schedule your family trip during the off season.
- Consider staying an extra day and making all the days at the park shorter (most young children do better with shorter days anyway).
- Prepare him through pictures and a promo video that talks about Disneyland.
- Walk him through what it will be like going to the front gate. Talk about all the people who will be walking around (such as at the mall). Talk about the characters that are at Disneyland, but tell him that he may only see a couple of them because they are not all there every day. (This is important for children in general, since they lock into what you have said. So if you said, "You will see Mickey, Ariel, and Pluto," your son may fixate on that and be very upset if he only gets to see Pocahontas!)
- If your town has "mini-carnival" type places, take your child there and explain how "Disneyland is like this, except bigger and noisier."
- Let him help pack his suitcase for your trip (start several days ahead of time).
- If additional family members are going, make sure to talk to them about your child's needs so that they will understand when he needs to "check out" from all the commotion.
- Remember: There is a fine line between preparing your child and talking the trip up too much. Be careful not to build it up

so much that when your child doesn't experience it the way you said it would be, he feels let down or that he has let you down. While you are there:

- Once of the biggest difficulties sensory-sensitive children have in a place like Disneyland is handling the noise and visual information coming at them all at once. Bring sunglasses and earplugs that your child can take in and out (bring an extra pair in case they get lost).
- When you get there, quickly identify a couple of spots that you and your child can use to escape to if he is feeling overwhelmed. Let him know that "you have staked out the place" and there are a couple of safe spots. The best quiet places are the higher-end restaurants. The two of you could just sit in a booth and order a drink for a break.
- Avoid the rides that involve a lot of movement along with visual and auditory input (tunnel-type rollercoasters). If your child insists, make sure to have the earplugs ready and a bag just in case he gets nauseous.
- Bring some sour, chewy candy so that if he starts to sweat and become nauseous, he can suck on something that will relieve some of this reaction.
- Make him suck on a lemon drop while waiting in line, but tell him to spit it out before getting on a ride.
- Consider bringing his favorite light jacket or sweatshirt (regardless of the weather). This could be his "escape" jacket for when he has had enough.
- If you can afford it, stay in one of the hotels on the grounds so you have a close place to take your child if he is done for the day, before everyone else is ready to go.
- Consider bringing some squeeze toys for him.

- Put all the "emergency gear" (sensory stuff) in a small backpack and let your child know what's in there.
- Make sure to continue some of the sensory exercises that he does daily at home.
- Have fun!!

Q. What can I do to help my child sit through a church service?

A. Look for services held at different times, such as Saturday night services, which tend to be more casual and shorter. Also consider the acoustics of your church. We typically don't pay attention to this but children who have SPD (auditory and vestibular processing sensitivities) "feel" the difference immediately. If possible, let the rest of the family go first, and you and your child follow a little later after the music that starts the service is over. Once seated, allow your child to wear earplugs or headphones during the service (ignore the looks; the powers above do not care). Make sure to sit in the back and let her take water breaks if she is having difficulty sitting still. If your child is tactilely defensive at all, wearing "dress clothes" may put her on edge before she even gets to church, so avoid the problem and dress her in comfortable clothes. Consider bringing a wedge cushion for her to sit on while in church, and let her bring a squeeze toy. You may also want to bring a small snack (but avoid crunchy foods).

Q. Are there any alternatives to play groups?

A. Try the "play date" model instead. First, call a few friends who have children your child's age and would be a good match for your child. Give the moms you talk to the option of staying or just dropping off their toddler. You may get a few more takers this way. Schedule a limited-time play date, of no more than an hour. Limit the number of toys each child can access and create physical boundaries for the play area so the children naturally play in the same area.

Have some "planned" activities set up that you know your child enjoys, such as crawling through tunnels, scooter games, water table play outside, Play-Doh play, or coloring, and make sure you have the materials on hand. Start with a gross motor activity that doesn't require a lot of interaction between two toddlers, such as riding toy cars, crawling through tunnels, and so on. Then move to more table or floor time activities that have some interaction—but don't expect a lot of interaction the first few times. Call it a success if the two toddlers played in the same area for any length of time. Use this model to expand your child's circle of friends.

A great resource for expanding your child's friendships through facilitated peer play is the video **Passport to Friendship**, by Hilary Baldi, M.A., and Deanne Detmers, M.A., of the Behavioral Intervention Association. This video was designed to help children with autism spectrum disorder make friends through play; however, many of the suggestions would help any child with difficulty in this area, especially children with SPD.

Q. How should I prepare my child for a Fourth of July party?

A. Depending on how sensitive your child is, your family may opt to leave the party before the fireworks are lit. If your decision is to stay, then make sure your child knows what is going to happen ahead of time. Explain to her that there will be fireworks at the party, but that mommy found a way to help her ears so she won't hear the loud noises but can still see the fireworks. You can try earplugs or headphones with a portable CD player. Be sure to talk to the host/hostess so that you know when they will start the fireworks.

Q. How do I plan a birthday party for my teenager who is easily overstimulated?

A. Pick an activity that your child will enjoy. For example, if swimming is his thing, make the party a swimming party. If he enjoys a treasure hunt, make the party a survivor/scavenger hunt party. When you sit down with your child to make the guest list, consider limiting the number of people who will attend. Encourage your child to only invite people he is comfortable around and that he thinks will have fun with. This is crucial. If there are other teens he wants to invite, but you suspect that they will think a "swimming" or a "survivor" themed party is not cool, then it is best not to invite them.

If the party is at your house, make sure you put decorations up a couple of days ahead of time so your child can get used to the changed space. If the party is at a strange location that you do not visit often, make sure you go there a couple of days before the party. This will give him a chance to get used to the new space and get a feel for himself in the new space before a bunch of people are surrounding him. Make sure you have activities planned out ahead of time because *nothing* is more anxiety provoking than a party where teenagers are standing in self-made groups with "no entrance" stamped across their faces.

You may want to stagger the invite times into two different groups of people. If there is a core group of friends that understand your child's difficulties in social situations, have them show up thirty minutes earlier than the next group. Thirty minutes is enough time to increase your child's comfort level with a few people so that he is more at ease when the other guests arrive. Also, you and your child can work into the party some planned "sensory breaks" from the group; if the party is at home, he can go into his room for awhile, and if it is at a restaurant or other facility, he can walk outside and do some push-ups against the wall or a similar activity.

Q. What are some general tips for helping my teenager in social situations, especially parties or large gatherings?

A. Consider putting your child on a "sensory diet" (described in Chapter 6) and have her do certain sensory activities that have a more calming effect right before a social event. Your child is old enough for you to teach her the "time out" social strategies that all of us adults use to regroup. These include going to the bathroom, even if you really don't have to; taking a walk and then returning to the social gathering; or just staring out the window as if you are admiring the flora of someone's home when you are actually just stealing a little downtime. Teach your child all your favorite strategies, such as "I have to make a call." When you are out with your child, try to verbalize all the internal talk you use to be successful in social situations.

Q. Should I enroll my child in a social skills training group?

A. Before you can make that decision, you want to take a look at the program curriculum. Is the curriculum teaching your child a menu of social niceties such as proper introductions, handshakes, and eye contact? Or is it an actual "social practice" time for your child to try these skills with peers in a protective environment? There are many "social skills" groups or even manuals that teach children techniques such as introducing themselves, but don't teach children how to *feel* more comfortable in social situations. These social nicety programs can inadvertently make a child seem even more odd to peers.

One of the best things you can do is to encourage social interaction in safe sensory environments that offer you some control and to prepare your child beforehand. For example, having a limited number of your child's friends over to your house for movie night is an unsafe sensory environment, whereas a trip to the movies is a nonsafe sensory environment because you cannot control the number of people, the smells, and the noise level. Visit public places during nonpeak times in order to acclimate your child to the situation. For example, do not plan a pizza night out on Friday or Saturday night between 5:00 and 8:00 pm.

Q. How do I stop my child from throwing temper tantrums in public?

A. Tantrums or meltdowns are more common in children with SPD than other children. They are a quick way to communicate "my nervous system has had enough" without using words. When any of us experience stress, finding the right words can be difficult. For children with SPD, this is even more pronounced, often they will go right to behavior to communicate their needs. As a parent, this can be very hard, but here are some key strategies that may help:

- Learn your child's triggers: when it happens, what time of day and where (after lunch? after a long car ride?).
- Learn the physical signs that occur right before a tantrum: yawning, scratching self, sucking thumb, whining, shaking his/her head, walking/dancing on tiptoes, asking repeatedly for food or drink, and other behaviors that might indicate your child's anxiety level is rising.
- Work out a sign that your child can give you when he can't maintain anymore, such as pulling on his ear, saying "air," or giving you a card that he carries in his pocket and places in your hand when he's overwhelmed. Make sure to establish rules around this—your child should understand that he can't do it all the time, only when he is feeling overwhelmed.

- Intervene at the first sign of a meltdown by taking your child to another room, and talking him through it to see if you can ease the difficulties. If you cannot solve the problem by talking, then it is time to go home. Do not force him through the negative situation; that is the part of the experience he will remember.

Q. How can we make going to a restaurant less of an ordeal?

A. Get the menu ahead of time so that your child is familiar with the choices. Make a game of choosing what item everyone will be eating. If going out to eat is a treat, then remember that this may not be the time to insist on healthy eating. Try to make going out to eat more about the social/family experience. Also, don't try to push for culinary exploration; if chicken fingers and fries is it, well, so be it. Even if you're going to a restaurant that doesn't take reservations, call ahead and explain that your child is easily over-whelmed. If you call a few days ahead of time, many restaurants will be understanding and try to accommodate you. Ask for a booth; rounded ones are best because they are usually in a corner and offer more visual blockage. Request a table that is away from high-traffic areas such as the front door or kitchen door.

If you cannot make arrangements with the restaurant, make sure you bring toys or other distractions to mitigate what may be an overwhelming situation for your child. Think of activities that will keep your child occupied. For example, bring a Styrofoam cup, a couple of markers, and a package of stickers to the restaurant. Tell your child that she gets to decorate her own cup. This is worth at least ten to fifteen minutes of activity.

Q. How can I help my child enjoy her friends' birthday parties?

A. This is a common concern for parents of children with SPD. The best advice is to choose parties wisely. There are many types of birthday parties—some are simple get-togethers, others are "events." If you know the party will be at a place with many blinking lights, choose not to attend. This kind of party equals a sure meltdown. A party that features an inflatable, bouncy house may be more appropriate, because your child can likely escape to her own place if she needs to.

Call the hosting parent ahead of time and ask if there is a place where your child can seek refuge if necessary. Also, make sure it is okay for you to stay. Most parents will be very understanding.

Go into the party knowing that you may have to leave early and/or may have to take sensory breaks. Make sure your child is aware that these options are available. Act immediately when you see that your child is becoming agitated or anxious; it is better to intervene at this age than have her memory of parties be linked with emotional disasters. Work out a hand signal that your child can give when she's at the end of her rope and needs your help. If your child chooses to stay in the bouncy house the entire time instead of participating in the other party activities, allow her to do this until she becomes more comfortable with the party routine.

Q. My child "freaks" at the thought of going to the dentist. What can I do?

A. You can employ a number of strategies to attempt to make the experience less traumatic. First, let your child know ahead of time what is going to happen at the dentist's office (even if he has been before). Use pictures to create a simple, positive story of going to the dentist and encourage him to re-create the dentist experience himself. Have him apply pressure with his fingers on his own mouth and let him know that is how it will feel. Have him open his own mouth wide while looking in the mirror and use his toothbrush to examine his own teeth. Tell him that is exactly what the dentist will do.

Once at the dentist, right before the dentist arrives (while your child is in the dentist's chair) apply deep pressure to his shoulders and back. Your child may like wearing a weighted vest or the X-ray apron during the visit. Use a timer that lets your child see how long the appointment is going to last, and let him hold a fidget toy or a weighted stuffed animal on his lap. Also consider letting your child wear Therapeutic Listening headphones, so he can still hear your voice through them. Last, ask the dentist to tell your child what is going to happen before he does each procedure.

Q. My child's grandparents give her gifts that she really likes, but her facial expression is either blank or pained. Her grandparents think she doesn't like the gifts. Is there anything I can do?

A. First explain to them that your child is experiencing sensory overload. Controlling her happy reactions to the gifts helps her control negative reactions to all the noises, visual stimuli, and people.

Here is another idea you might want to try. Practice Christmas: For one week leading up to the Christmas holidays, wrap up your child's used toys and have her practice unwrapping them and being happy about the gift. Teach her to say things like, "I love this," "This is cool," and "Thank you." Parents who have tried this report seeing a positive difference in their child's reactions, which makes everybody's experience more positive.

Chapter 12 | TOUCHY TOPICS

- Why does my child who is tactilely defensive touch herself inappropriately?
- Is there anything I can do to decrease my child's desire to touch herself?
- If my child touches herself inappropriately at school, how can I get her to stop?
- Why does my child play with his saliva and always have his fingers in his mouth?
- My one-and-a-half-year-old child is still eating baby food because he gags on solid food. Is this linked to some of his other sensory behaviors?
- Why does my child eat dirt and lick odd things like rocks, metal fences, and paint if I don't watch her?
- The minute my child gets home, she sheds her clothes. What can I do?
- My child is often constipated and says his "butt hurts." Is this linked to his sensory defensive issues?
- Why does my child bite himself on the arm when we are out in public, and how can I stop it?
- Why does my child have to strip off all his clothes before he can go poop?
- Can the onset of puberty trigger SPD issues that my child had when she was younger?
- Could regular bedwetting in an eight-year-old child be due to SPD?
- My twelve-year-old child often smells bad because she will not bathe. What can I do?

Q. Why does my child who is tactilely defensive touch herself inappropriately?

A. It is not uncommon for children who are tactilely defensive to seek out intense kinds of input. The input your child is receiving from masturbating is intense and rhythmic in nature; thus it has a calming, integrating effect on the body. Children who are sensitive to light touch will often seek out deep-pressure (proprioceptive) input since it has a calming effect on the body.

Q. Is there anything I can do to decrease my child's desire to touch herself?

A. Most children touch themselves, at least in exploration. Your child may have an increased drive toward this type of stimulation because of its intense input to her nervous system. Try getting her on a regular brushing program (see Chapter 6) coupled with a lot of deep-pressure-type input, such as jumping on a trampoline, being squeezed between two bean bags, or wearing a weighted vest.

Q. If my child touches herself inappropriately at school, how can I get her to stop?

A. First, have a sensory integration evaluation done on your child, because chances are there are other sensory issues connected to this behavior. Consult the occupational therapist to get your child on a regular brushing program and a program that offers increased opportunities for deep-pressure input to other parts of her body. This program often results in less inappropriate touching since the child gets intense sensory stimulation from another source, such as intense head massage or increased input to the jaw through crunchy food or a therapeutic vibrator. Then talk to your child about when and where she can touch herself. The key is that she understands why she is doing it and that she isn't "bad" or "misbehaving," but that her body desires intense sensory input. Tell her that she can do that in the privacy of her own room.

Q. Why does my child play with his saliva and always have his fingers in his mouth?

A. Your child is most likely seeking increased oral stimulation. Children who are hyposensitive to oral stimulation will often have their fingers in their mouths because they are seeking increased amounts of oral stimulation. To help your child stop playing with his saliva, provide him with increased amounts of oral input. Try the following strategies:

- Let him use a battery-operated toothbrush (they are not as intense as the electric ones and kids seem to like them better).
- Offer him textured snacks, such as popcorn, apples, and gummy worms (a limited amount).
- Practice oral-motor exercises.
- Use a chewy tube.
- Encourage blowing bubbles, blowing on whistles, and sucking through a crazy straw.
- Try letting him suck on Lemon Head candies; they are sweet and sour enough to make anyone pucker.

Q. My one-and-a-half-year-old child is still eating baby food because he gags on solid food. Is this linked to some of his other sensory behaviors?

A. Your pediatrician should check to see if your child has ENT or GI problems that could be related to his SPD, as both reflux and sensory issues can contribute to gagging. A thorough evaluation may include a "modified barium swallow study" to be sure his chewing and swallowing mechanisms are working properly. In order to determine if the gagging is related to sensory processing issues, Catherine Leavitt, a feeding and swallowing expert, suggests that the therapist would want to answer the following questions:

- Does the child gag on pieces of all textures or just certain ones of a particular size or taste?
- Does he chew his food up enough to mash it?
- Does he have a hypersensitive gag?
- Does he reject the food just by looking at it—especially if it is a new food? Or does he wait until he tries the food and actually gags as a result of the texture?
- Does the child use the gagging behavior to manipulate parents out of eating so he can have a bottle?
- How did the child score on the oral sensitivity portion of the Infant/Toddler Sensory Profile?
- Where do his sensitivities begin: his mouth, jaw, or hairline?
- What other items does the child put into his mouth?

Once the therapist determines there is a sensory problem that causes all or part of the gagging behavior, treatment can begin. The treatment would most likely involve desensitization of the sensitive areas of the face and/or inside the mouth and working with textures. It is extremely important to get started quickly with treatment while the child is still young, so the gagging behavior (regardless of its source) is not reinforced for long periods of time.

Q. Why does my child eat dirt and lick odd things like rocks, metal fences, and paint if I don't watch her?

A. Most children at a young age will put objects in their mouths as a way of tactile discovery, which is a very important stage. Past that age (approximately 24 months), licking inedible objects may be a sign that your child is hyposensitive to oral stimulation and is seeking out intense taste, tactile, and proprioceptive input. Try letting your child use a battery-operated toothbrush and offer him textured snacks, such as popcorn, apples, and gummy worms (a limited amount).

Other strategies include practicing oral-motor exercises, using a chewy tube, and encouraging your child to blow bubbles, blow on whistles, and suck through a crazy straw. Make sure to watch your child closely because of health concerns; many children who are hyposensitive lick things like metal and paint that can (obviously) be detrimental to their health.

Q. The minute my child gets home, she sheds her clothes. What can I do?

A. It sounds like your child is tactically defensive and may be holding it together all day at school, but looking forward to the moment when she can literally strip the irritation from her body. Provide her with some calming-type input, such as lotion and massage to her arms, brushing, and deep pressure. Tell her that she can have an "outside" set of clothes that she wears to school, and then a "home wardrobe" that she gets to choose. I suggest things like extra-large t-shirts, large boxer shorts, and anything big with soft cotton-type fabrics.

Q. My child is often constipated and says his "butt hurts." Is this linked to his sensory defensive issues?

A. Your child's sensory defensiveness may be contributing to his constipation. First look at his diet. If his sensory defensiveness results in him being a picky eater, he may avoid certain types of foods that contain fiber, which would ease his constipation. His defensiveness may also mean that he is sensitive to bowel movements (they may be especially painful if he is constipated) and he may be reflexively contracting his anus, causing back up and compounding the problem. Children who are sensory defensive are also prone to high anxiety, which can be linked to constipation.

Try to change the experience into something positive. Make it less about producing something, and more about relaxation, sitting alone, or listening to music. If your child needs you in the bathroom, play a game with him like "What am I thinking of?" (animal, plant, etc.), rather than just sitting there. Talk to your child's pediatrician about using a fiber solution, and try a number of different fruits and vegetables to see if there are some he will try.

Q. Why does my child bite himself on the arm when we are out in public, and how can I stop it?

A. Most likely your child is feeling overwhelmed and doesn't know how to deal with it. The biting gives his jaw and arm increased proprioceptive input, which is very integrating. Besides using it as a sensory strategy, he may be trying to communicate that he is overwhelmed and afraid. This is one of those times when you are going to have to be your child's sensory detective. Make sure you record exactly what public situation the biting takes place in. This way you can limit his exposure to those situations. Also, utilize strategies for oral input and proprioceptive input for the hands.

Q. Why does my child have to strip off all his clothes before he can go poop?

A. Without knowing your child, there are two possibilities that he may be experiencing: under-responsiveness or over-responsiveness from tactile/proprioceptive input. If he is under-responsive to sensory input, it may take more concentration than normal for his nervous system to register internal processing such as a bowel movement. Removing his clothes allows him to register that information and go to the bathroom easier.

If he is over-responsive to sensory input, it may be overwhelming for him to process the bowel movement as well as take in the sensory input from his clothes. (Some children who are over-responsive remove all their clothes, turn off the light, and demand complete silence so they can have a bowel movement.) Since pooping is a private experience, you should respect whichever strategies your child needs to employ. This may not be possible in public places, but, in general, most children get beyond this once they have the proper sensory input.

Q. Can the onset of puberty trigger SPD issues that my child had when she was younger?

A. As we all know, puberty brings on changes in hormone levels in the body. Hormones have a direct effect on the neurochemicals that drive nervous-system processing. So it makes sense that hormone levels would exacerbate underlying nervous-system processing difficulties. Your child may have been through sensory therapy as a child, and now it is time to talk to her about her body. You would have had to do this anyway when she reached puberty. Now you just have another layer to add to the discussion.

Make your child newly aware of how her sensory defensiveness is affecting how she feels. She may have to incorporate some of the strategies that worked before, such as the Wilbarger Deep Pressure program, to help her manage her defensiveness during these years of changes. The difference is that this time it is imperative that your child learn how to implement these strategies herself.

Q. Could regular bedwetting in an eight-year-old child be due to SPD?

A. Possibly. Your child's nervous system may be having difficulty processing the information that his bladder is full while he is sleeping. There are many steps that your child's nervous system must take in order to avoid wetting the bed. He must register the internal sensory stimulation that his bladder is full, his brain must wake him up, and he must quickly orient himself in a dark room and get to the bathroom in time.

In this case, it is beneficial to use some common parenting strategies that are not necessarily sensory based that will help your child to not wet the bed. Decrease liquids for a few hours before bedtime, wake your child up at a set time every night to use the bathroom (eventually you can use a musical alarm), and make sure he has a lighted path to the bathroom. In conjunction with above-mentioned strategies, you can also increase proprioceptive and tactile input to help with sensory registration.

Q. My twelve-year-old child often smells bad because she will not bathe. What can I do?

A. If the showering issue is new, it may be related to puberty. It is important to discuss with your child other people's perceptions and reassure her that you are open to finding alternative ways for her to bathe herself.

Try to address the underlying sensory defensiveness. This may be a good time to visit an occupational therapist, as it is often easier for a teenager to listen to an outside person than listen to a parent. Sensory strategies need to be coupled with behavior modification. Agree upon a rule whereby your child takes a bath or shower once per week (early Sunday evening, for example) for a limited period of time. Other days she can cleanse herself using a washcloth. Try using different textures of washcloth to find one that does not trigger her sensory defensiveness.

Chapter 13

THE ADULT YEARS

- Why don't I know any adults with sensory processing disorder?
- Do children who have SPD grow up to be adults with "issues"?
- If a child doesn't receive therapy, can he "outgrow" SPD?
- Now that my child has been diagnosed with SPD, I realize that I have the same issues. Is it too late to get help?
- Once I start doing sensory integration therapy, how long will it take to see changes?
- I suffer from severe anxiety attacks, and I am sensitive to touch and certain noises. Should I get evaluated for SPD?
- Could my clumsiness be due to Sensory Processing Disorder?
- What type of sensory processing difficulty has the biggest impact on adults?
- What are the characteristics of adults who have Sensory Processing Disorder?
- How do you test for sensory processing disorder in an adult?
- Does the aging process affect our sensory processing abilities?
- Can doing sensory-integrative types of activities slow the aging process?

Q. Why don't I know any adults with sensory processing disorder?

A. You do. At least 5 percent of the population has sensory processing difficulties, and many children become adults without getting any help. The reason you may not be aware of a friend or colleague who has SPD is that as an adult, a person can choose to stay clear of sensory experiences that are uncomfortable. No one will make them go to a noisy birthday party, or eat oatmeal with lumps, or wear polyester. By the time most people reach adulthood, they have learned to work around or with their various difficulties. Those with SPD are no different.

For example, the adult with auditory defensiveness will probably not be found at places where there is loud music. The adult with tactile issues will probably not be a chef, since this often requires touching "icky" stuff. With that said, adults with SPD who have not sought help or learned strategies to help themselves will continue to have difficulties in social situations, motor and vocational activities, and may also have difficulties in intimate relationships due to issues with touch.

Q. Do children who have SPD grow up to be adults with "issues"?

A. First of all, this *is* the 21st century, so you are not an adult unless you have some "issues." The real question is: How do these issues affect your life, and how do you choose to deal with them?

The advantage of a child who has been diagnosed with SPD is that he will get just the right amount of input in a safe therapy environment. This gives the child's nervous system an opportunity to strengthen some of those weaker connections as well as learn to adjust behavior to stimuli that may be perceived as threatening. Most important, the child with SPD who gets treatment will grow up with a better understanding of his body and brain. He will most likely learn strategies and behavioral adaptations that will help him become a more successful adult.

Q. If a child doesn't receive therapy, can he "outgrow" SPD?

A. Because SPD is due to underlying neurological difficulties, if a child's sensory processing is not addressed, the chance that she will simply "outgrow" the disorder is slim. If a child does not receive help for sensory processing difficulties, the problems will most likely become magnified or the child will find ways to withdraw from situations where her sensory systems could be "under attack." Increased reactivity and isolation will both have negative impacts upon your child into adulthood.

Q. Now that my child has been diagnosed with SPD, I realize that I have the same issues. Is it too late to get help?

A. When learning about sensory processing difficulties in another person, it is not uncommon to identify sensory issues in yourself that you may have attributed to a lack of coordination, fear of heights, depression, or extreme shyness. Most important, it is *never* too late to help your nervous system work more effectively. Sometimes, therapists who are taking advanced training for sensory integration will realize that *they* have sensory processing problems that are impacting their lives. They will use the principles of sensory integration therapy to help themselves or seek direct therapy from another therapist. Also, many parents of children treated for SPD become aware of their own sensory issues and use tactile, auditory, visual, or vestibular treatment strategies assigned to their children on themselves, and see improvements.

Q. Once I start doing sensory integration therapy, how long will it take to see changes?

A. As an adult, you will most likely notice changes immediately. Participating in sensory integration therapy is similar to any other kind of treatment regime you may embark on. Results will depend on how closely you follow the treatment and how consistent you are with therapy. Usually, as adults our therapy is completely voluntary and we are seeking change, so we are more likely to participate in some of the activities, even if there is some discomfort in the beginning.

Q. I suffer from severe anxiety attacks, and I am sensitive to touch and certain noises. Should I get evaluated for SPD?

A. Yes, see an occupational therapist and be evaluated for sensory processing disorder, especially sensory modulation disorder. Your anxiety could be linked to sensory defensiveness. When you are particularly sensitive to certain stimuli, this can cause you to have increased anxiety because you can't control when your nervous system is going to be bombarded by uncomfortable touch or noise. Anxiety is often a fear of the unknown, and may be a manifestation of feeling out of control.

Q. Could my clumsiness be due to Sensory Processing Disorder?

A. Yes, it could. You can think of motor planning capabilities as a spectrum. There is the person whose nervous system is so well integrated that it allows for incredible natural motor planning abilities, such as the professional football player who leaps in the air to catch a football while running at breakneck speed and hits the ground in full stride, or the ballerina who does a pirouette, or your best friend who can replicate every new dance step just by watching it once. At the other end of the spectrum are people whose motor planning takes much more cognitive energy as well as practice. But practice only gets you so far when you have motor planning difficulties. For example, if your visual-vestibular system is not working well, it can cause you to feel insecure about your body and especially insecure when your body has to react to a moving object, such as a baseball.

Q. What type of sensory processing difficulty has the biggest impact on adults?

A. Sensory Modulation Disorder seems to have the most serious impact on the success of adults. It can cause a person to have difficulty managing reactions to incoming stimuli in the many different environments that are necessary to live a full life as an adult. It has a direct impact on a person's social and emotional well-being.

Q. What are the characteristics of adults who have Sensory Processing Disorder?

A. Here is a short list of symptoms and reaction characteristics for adolescents and adults with SPD. Keep in mind that if you fit one or two of these, you probably do not have SPD; it is only when a number of these are present or extreme that you may want to seek an evaluation.

Signs of Sensory Modulation Difficulties

- Bothered by certain clothing materials, such as tags, seams, and turtlenecks
- Uncomfortable with the touch component of relationships, such as snuggling or massages
- Seems over- or under-reactive to pain

- Bothered by light touch and would prefer to be the "toucher" rather than the "touchee"
- Avoids touching anything that is messy, such as an art project or certain foods
- Has extremes in food tastes, either extremely bland or extremely spicy
- Tendency toward eating-disorder-type behaviors, or has sensitivities to eating
- Needs to sleep with multiple heavy blankets
- Avoids escalators
- Gags when exposed to certain smells, such as perfume, food, or body odors
- Extreme fear of heights
- Constantly fiddling with anything they can get their hands on, even when they know it is socially inappropriate
- Extreme motion sickness, cannot ride in the back seat of cars
- Chain smokes
- Avoids social situations with lots of people
- Overly distracted by noises others do not notice, such as computers or air conditioners
- Unusually uncomfortable when there is a change in acoustics, such as in old churches or auditoriums
- Turns to alcohol or drugs to modulate self

Signs of Sensory Discrimination Difficulties

- Uses eyesight instead of touch for typical activities, such as getting dressed or finding things in a purse
- Struggles with following symbolic information, such as traffic signs and warning symbols

- Has a complete lack of sense of direction, gets lost in familiar neighborhoods, can even get "turned around" in a grocery store
- Has difficulty adjusting voice volume appropriate to setting
- Must be completely isolated from distractions to complete any cognitive task
- Fixates easily on one activity, forgoing other things in the environment
- Has noticeable difficulties with articulation and enunciating words clearly
- Has difficulty using the appropriate amount of pressure when picking up objects (breaks things), hugging others, or shaking hands (limp or crushing)
- Is not able to easily distinguish different tastes and smells

Signs of Sensory-Based Motor Disorders

- Is clumsy and accident prone, bumping into people and things
- Can't remember left from right
- Has fine motor difficulties, including difficulties with tying, buttoning, manipulating small parts, as well as handwriting
- Favors sedentary activities, avoids sports and other physical activities
- Unusually low endurance for physical activity
- Must talk self through motor tasks
- When trying to perform multistep tasks, loses place and forgets next task

Q. How do you test for sensory processing disorder in an adult?

A. Adults are usually able to give plenty of feedback on a questionnaire and also give good information about themselves as a child, so those methods are preferred. Also, the Winnie Dunn Sensory Profile (Adult Adolescent Version) and allows the therapist to pinpoint the sensory areas that are impacting a person's day-to-day life the most. The occupational therapist will also do some clinical observation to see how a person will perform certain activities.

Q. Does the aging process affect our sensory processing abilities?

A. Yes, just as an immature nervous system has trouble processing sensory information, so does an aging nervous system. However, it is not just the aging process that impacts our nervous system but the decrease in activities that challenges our sensory-nervous system, especially the core senses—the vestibular, proprioceptive, and tactile systems. Here is a list of activities that will help keep our basic sensory systems in working condition for a longer period of time:

- Riding a bike, even mountain biking
- Walks, especially on rugged terrain
- Rock climbing, or walking on gently sloping rocks
- Learning a new dance
- Ball sports, especially ones that require coordination related to a moving ball
- Lifting weights
- Downhill or cross-country skiing
- Sledding
- Rolling around on the floor with your kids
- Hiking
- Karate
- Horseback riding

- A basic training type of workout, where you have to crawl on the ground before climbing a wall
- All activities that challenge your balance system and improve core strength, such as yoga—the key is to move your head and body into positions other than sitting, standing, and lying

Q. Can doing sensory-integrative types of activities slow the aging process?

A. Not much research has been done related to whether sensory integration therapy slows the aging process, although there is anecdotal evidence to suggest that it may be true. There is research on the positive impact that weight-bearing training (which is a proprioceptive activity) has on reversing lost capabilities. In addition, research shows that balance retraining (a vestibular activity) can reduce the number of times an aging person falls.

Chapter 14

SPD AND OTHER DISORDERS

- Is SPD a sign of autism?
- Is SPD worse and more common in children with autism?
- What are the most common sensory difficulties in children with autism?
- What are "stemming" behaviors?
- My child just started displaying stemming behaviors. What should I do?
- If my child has just been diagnosed with autism, is it better to pursue sensory integration therapy or an applied behavior analysis program?
- Does my child have Sensory Processing Disorder or attention deficit-hyperactive disorder?
- What are the differences in symptoms between SPD and ADHD or ADD?
- Since my child starting taking medication for ADHD, his sensory-seeking behaviors have decreased. Does that mean his sensory issues have been resolved?
- My two-year-child has been diagnosed with fragile X syndrome. Are sensory processing difficulties common in this population?
- Would an autism teaching program be a match for my child with fragile X?
- Where can I get more information specific to the sensory and social issues related to fragile X?
- Are there other diagnoses that are known to have a sensory processing component?

Q. Is SPD a sign of autism?

A. Sensory processing disorder and autism are separate diagnoses, and it would certainly be a reach to say that because a child has sensory processing difficulties, he is autistic. With that said, difficulties with sensory processing along with communication delays are often what parents see in a young child who will later be given a diagnosis of autism spectrum disorder. A study conducted by Dr. Lucy Jane Miller, a leading researcher on SPD, showed that more than 75 percent of children with autism or Asperger's syndrome have significant symptoms of Sensory Processing Disorder. There are several additional characteristics of a child with autism spectrum disorder (ASD) in addition to sensory sensitivities. Here are some of the hallmarks of ASD:

- Does not appear to want to engage others in activities or interests
- Lacks purposeful, expressive language
- Uses echolaic speech (repeats words or lines from movies that are not part of the conversation)
- Seems to want to be alone
- Has unpredictable reactions to any change
- May not appear to enjoy physical contact such as holding/cuddling
- Makes little/no eye contact
- Typical teaching methods do not seem to work
- Continuously spins objects
- Inappropriate attachments to objects
- Apparent over-sensitivity or under-sensitivity to pain
- Lacks fear of dangerous situations
- Extreme physical over-activity or under-activity
- Uneven gross/fine motor skills
- May seem to not hear people who are talking to them

Early signs of autism:

- At six months does not smile
- At twelve months lacks babbling, pointing, or other gestures
- Does not use single words by age sixteen months, or lacks the use of two-word phrases by twenty-four months
- Development regresses, with the loss of language or social skills

Q. Is SPD worse and more common in children with autism?

A. It is very common for a child with autism to also have SPD. It is reported that more than ninety percent of children with Autism Spectrum Disorder have sensory processing difficulties. The level of SPD severity varies in children with autism, as it does in all children with sensory processing difficulties. However, children with autism may have additional difficulties communicating to others what sensations are uncomfortable and scary, versus satisfying and calming. When individuals do not have the ability to communicate, they often use behavior to let others know what they think about something. Many children with autism use behavior to communicate fears, which people may misinterpret. Communication difficulties can easily exacerbate the severity of behavioral reactions to sensory input.

Q. What are the most common sensory difficulties in children with autism?

A. Although children with autism battle with many sensory issues, the most commonly reported are sensitivities to touch, auditory input, and smell. However, it is safe to say that most children with an autism spectrum diagnosis also display difficulties in motor-based sensory areas, such as praxis. Many children with a diagnosis of autism try to avoid touch, especially unexpected touch. Sometimes this is interpreted as not enjoying physical contact or avoiding people, but it is actually because they perceive light touch as painful, resulting in a fear response. Many of these individuals will go to great lengths to avoid this kind of sensory input. They may enjoy or even seek out deep pressure since it has a calming effect.

When trying to help a child with autism become more accustomed to different textures or unexpected touch, it helps to pair that input with proprioceptive input (deep pressure). Sometimes a short-term intense brushing program can go a long way toward desensitizing a child. Parents will often report that their child with autism also has sensitivities to noises. Sensory integration therapy can help a child process auditory input more effectively, as well as teach the child how to cope with unexpected noises. There are activities you can do with your child to help him "get used" to noise in a fun way.

Q. What are "stemming" behaviors?

A. Stemming behaviors are repetitive behaviors such as handclapping, rocking, and even biting. It could even be actions such as opening and closing a door or turning a light on and off. Stemming behaviors are often seen in children with an autism diagnosis. They can be a way of organizing themselves when they are over stimulated or arousing themselves when they are under stimulated. They may also be how that child communicates fear, excitement, confusion, or even anger. It is important to note when stemming behaviors occur, what precedes them, as well as if certain sensory input, such as vestibular or proprioceptive input, decreases the occurrence of the behaviors.

Q. My child just started displaying stemming behaviors. What should I do?

A. Never ignore stemming behaviors because they may be your child's way of communicating that something is wrong or organizing himself. Also, unless the behavior is harmful to your child or anyone else, don't try to stop the behavior immediately. First, figure out why your child may be engaged in the behavior and what alternative behavior you can teach him that may be less distracting to others. Consider if there have been any changes in your child's life that could be distressing. Keep in mind that for a child with autism, behaviors can be triggered by minor changes. Also, try the stemming behavior yourself and see how it makes you feel. This may give you a better idea of what your child is getting out of the behavior and thus why he may be engaging in it. For example, if you flap your hands in front of your eyes, you are stimulating the proprioceptive sensors in your wrists; if you watch your hands, you will stimulate your visual-vestibular system because fixating the eyes on a rapidly moving object stimulates this response.

Q. If my child has just been diagnosed with autism, is it better to pursue sensory integration therapy or an applied behavior analysis program?

A. It is important to get your child on an applied behavior analysis (ABA) program, so that she will learn how to learn. In other words, she will actually learn how to respond to input—whether it be a gesture, a picture, or a verbal request. This will set your child up to participate in academics and socialization. ABA programs are simply the application of the science of behavior and are designed according to this simple premise: a stimulus is presented, then there is a response, and then there is a consequence. For example, if you have two different colored blocks present and you ask a child to point to the blue block (this is the stimulus), she points to the blue block (that is the response). Then you say, "Yes that is the blue block. . . good job" (that is the consequence). If she had pointed to the green block, the consequence would be to show her the blue block and ensure success the next time you ask the question. ABA programs break skills down and teach children to respond to requests. Also, ABA has been morphing, and many practitioners are delivering the same instruction encompassed in naturalistic activities such as play.

It is imperative that your child's sensory processing needs are addressed in addition to the ABA program. Your child should be evaluated by an occupational therapist who has worked with children who have autism spectrum disorder. Make sure you or the occupational therapist share the report with the behaviorist in charge of your child's ABA program. See if the ABA program team and occupational therapist can meet for some joint sessions with your child. It is important that the ABA program team works with your child's occupational therapist so they have a clear picture of her sensory-motor weaknesses and strengths and can gear their instruction accordingly. Conversely, after your child's occupational therapist works with the ABA team, she or he will have a clear idea of some of the learning objectives of the ABA team.

Q. Does my child have Sensory Processing Disorder or attention deficit-hyperactive disorder?

A. These two disorders can look alike. A child with ADHD may have a secondary diagnosis of SPD. However, the two are different and look different to trained clinicians. For instance, children with SPD seek activity that is directly related to the sensation they crave, and when they get the sensation they need, there are changes in attention, restlessness, activity levels, and self-control. It may take time to see the long-term changes, but the right input should have immediate effects on the child with SPD. On the flip side, children with ADHD may appear to jump from activity to activity with no clear pattern of seeking a particular input, nor will they appear to avoid specific inputs.

Q. What are the differences in symptoms between SPD and ADHD or ADD?

A. As said before, these disorders can look very similar. There is not much variety in the symptoms; rather, it is the fundamental driver of the behaviors and how the behaviors change based on sensory input that is different for each disorder. For example, children with either disorder can appear very disorganized, be impatient, and have difficulty attending, as well as seem disinterested and uncooperative. However, sensory input helps the child with SPD become more organized, more patient, and better focused. It is important to keep in mind that children with ADHD may have sensory processing difficulties in addition to ADHD.

Q. Since my child starting taking medication for ADHD, his sensory-seeking behaviors have decreased. Does that mean his sensory issues have been resolved?

A. Although the medication may have tempered some of his sensory-seeking behaviors, his nervous system has not learned to process the information differently. Rather, it has been given an additive (the medication) that has altered the neurochemicals in the brain that directly impact his nervous system's function. In your son's case, the impact has been a positive one. However, as a parent and a medical professional, I encourage parents to view medications that alter neurochemistry as temporary and to look to more long-term solutions, such as increased sensory processing abilities linked with behavioral modifications both at school and at home. With that in mind, I would recommend continuing to implement sensory strategies throughout your son's day as well as behavioral modifications.

Q. My two-year-old child has been diagnosed with fragile X syndrome. Are sensory processing difficulties common in this population?

A. It is very common for children with fragile X syndrome to have sensory processing difficulties. A child with fragile X syndrome is very likely to display sensory overresponsivity to varying stimuli, which leads to a state of hyperarousal. Difficulties with hyperarousal have been well documented in children with fragile X syndrome. When your son is hyperaroused, you are likely to see some behaviors that can be alarming or annoying. These behaviors could include perseverating speech (sounds like a broken record), hand-flapping, biting, repetitive motor actions, as well as a marked decrease in eye contact. (Note: When children with fragile X are not overaroused, they exhibit eye contact and are very socially engaging.)

Q. Would an autism teaching program be a good match for my child with fragile X?

A. According to the experts, children with fragile X typically have different learning styles than children who have an autism spectrum diagnosis. A program geared toward children with autism that utilizes discrete trial, forward chaining, and TEACH methods works great for children with autism but may not be a good match for your child. The experts on fragile X emphasize that children with fragile X learn much differently than children with autism. Children with fragile X tend to be what experts refer to as "Gestalt" learners or whole learners. Therefore, they need to see and understand the whole activity or picture to be motivated to complete the parts.

With that said, there are ABA (applied behavior analysis) approaches such as Pivot Response Training and Whole Task Learning that work well for children with fragile X. Also, consider some of the relationship-based programs for children with fragile X, such as RDI (Relationship Development Intervention) as well as Greenspan's Floor Time because these programs emphasize social-sensory components of developmental learning. It is important that you are aware of your child's learning style and make others on your child's team aware of this style, and specifically issues related to hyperarousal.

Q. Where can I get more information specific to the sensory and social issues related to fragile X?

A. National Fragile X Foundation

Developmental FX: The Developmental and Fragile X Resource Centre co-founded by Tracy Murnan Stackhouse, MA, OTR, and Sarah Scharfenaker, MA, CCC-SLP. They are both very knowledge-able and speak internationally on topics related to fragile X. www.developmentalfx.com

The Mind Institute in Sacramento California is doing a lot of research concerning fragile X syndrome.

University of Denver—Fisher Early Learning Center

Q. Are there other diagnoses that are known to have a sensory processing component?

A. Yes, there are a number of different diagnoses that commonly include sensory processing issues, such as:

- Nonverbal learning disability
- Asperger's syndrome
- Schizophrenia

- Bipolar disorder
- Obsessive-compulsive disorder
- Drug and alcohol addiction
- Depression (sometimes SPD can lead to this due to social difficulties)

Chapter 15

SPECIAL POPULATIONS

- Are premature babies at increased risk for SPD?
- Do hospitals consider the sensory issues when a child is born premature?
- What are signs of sensory processing difficulties in a premature infant?
- Is there a connection between learning disabilities and sensory processing difficulties?
- My child is in special education due to speech and language difficulties but has also been identified as "gifted and talented." Can he be both?
- Is there a link between sensory issues and fetal alcohol syndrome?
- Will sensory integration therapy help a child with impulsive behaviors?
- If we are adopting internationally, should we be concerned about SPD?
- Are specific sensory issues more prevalent in children from certain countries?
- We just adopted our child from an orphanage in China. If she's sixteen months old and can't walk, should we be concerned that she has motor difficulties?
- If my internationally adopted child has some sensory and motor issues, does that mean she has SPD?
- Is there any link between children with reactive attachment disorder and SPD?
- Is there anything I can do to help my adopted child "undo" her first year in the orphanage?

Q. Are premature babies at increased risk for SPD?

A. Research indicates that children who were born premature are at increased risk of having sensory processing difficulties. When a child is born premature, she is more likely to have an underdeveloped or immature nervous system, compounded by the fact that she is placed in the ICU and may have to undergo intrusive medical procedures. This is the polar opposite of the child who is born full term, put on his mother's belly, and welcomed with soothing tactical and proprioceptive input.

Think about the sensory-safe world that an infant is in before entering the world. In the womb an infant spends its time in the dark, curled up, surrounded by nutrient-rich, protective fluid, while listening to the mother's soothing heartbeat layered with soft sounds from the outside world. This sensory-protected environment lays the foundation for nervous system growth during this stage of life. The developing infant's nervous system requires this precious time to develop the neural connections that will allow it to process all the sensory information that it will encounter in a more complicated world. So if an infant enters the "sensory loud" world too early, her nervous system may not be prepared to handle it.

Q. Do hospitals consider the sensory issues when a child is born premature?

A. Most neonatal intensive care units in hospitals are becoming very aware of the sensory sensitivities of premature infants. Although most hospitals try to minimize the amount of stimulation that a premature infant receives, they cannot control all the noises, lights, and invasive touching and moving that goes on in the medical care of these infants. NICUs are including occupational therapists as part of their primary team who consult with the medical staff, as well as the parents, on ways to provide a sensory-soothing environment for premature infants or children born with other difficulties.

Q. What are signs of sensory processing difficulties in a premature infant?

A. Each baby is, of course, totally unique, but in general preemies with sensory processing difficulties tend to exhibit the following signs:

- Oral defensiveness due to feeding tubes, respirators, and suctioning
- Have either high or low tone in their muscles
- High sensitivity to sensory input
- Defensive protective reflex active longer than usual (startle easily)
- Tend toward extremes; either highly distractible/active or quiet/sleep often
- Vision problems

If you have a premature infant, ask if the hospital will put you in contact with an occupational therapist so you understand and meet your child's sensory needs while avoiding sensory overload. For example, discuss the best ways to position him in his crib and for feedings, how to caress him with firm rather than light touch, how intensely to rock him, and so on. Many parents have found infant massage to be very calming to premature infants. The most important thing to remember is to control the amount of sensory input your infant gets in those first months since his nervous system is less mature than an infant born full term.

Q. Is there a connection between learning disabilities and sensory processing difficulties?

A. Yes. Jean Ayres, the founder of sensory integration theory, was driven toward this by her own learning disability. Sensory Integration International as well as other institutions that are devoted to studying sensory integration estimate that as many as 70 percent of school-aged children with learning disabilities have some degree of sensory integration difficulties. Many children who have learning disabilities often have a history of other issues that can impact nervous system development, such as premature birth, some developmental delays, and poor motor coordination.

Improving a child's sensory processing can go a long way toward improving academic success. This is accomplished by targeting skills that are foundational for learning, such as visual skills, visual-motor skills, auditory processing skills, balance and motor skills, and tactical-proprioceptive skills. For example, if a child has visual skills difficulties, it is likely that she has a hard time reading or copying from a board. A child with auditory processing deficits will have difficulty interpreting what is heard or filtering out background noises so she can focus on the pertinent information from the current lesson.

Q. My child is in special education due to speech and language difficulties but has also been identified as "gifted and talented." Can he be both?

A. Yes, and bravo to your child's school. It is important that schools realize that a child may struggle in one area while still possessing gifts in other areas. These students can become the most frustrated since they are bright and possess strengths but, depending on the school and the teachers involved, may or may not be recognized for their talents. The fact that your child is getting special education services and will also receive special programming under "gifted and talented" speaks to the fact that the school recognizes that children learn differently.

Q. Is there a link between sensory issues and fetal alcohol syndrome?

A. The new terminology is *fetal alcohol spectrum disorder* (FASD), which refers to a range of neurological impairments that can affect a child who has been exposed to alcohol in the womb. Since FASD does affect the nervous system, there is a strong possibility it will manifest in sensory processing difficulties. The degree to which a child's neurological system is impacted depends on a number of factors, including how much alcohol was consumed and at what point during the pregnancy the alcohol was consumed, because there are key times when neurological structures are being formed. The severity of these issues is seen in a child's cognitive, motor, and behavior capabilities. The specific sensory issues that a child will face are related to the amount of neurological impairment. But in general, a child with fetal alcohol spectrum disorder is more sensory sensitive than other children and reacts more impulsively to input from the environment.

Q. Will sensory integration therapy help a child with impulsive behaviors?

A. You can consult an occupational therapist and consider doing a "trial" run of sensory integration therapy. If the problem is sensory based, your child would most likely benefit from a consistent behavior plan that is carried out at home and at school along with sensory strategies. A social story detailing what behavior is acceptable and how others respond to the impulsive behavior will help your child understand how his behavior is perceived and give him new behaviors he can use to get others' attention or calm himself.

Also, when your child becomes agitated, he may need a calming break, such as sitting in a bean bag chair for up to five minutes. Use a Visual Time Timer (timetimer.com) so that he can see how much time he has in the calming space or engage in a sensory activity before returning to what he was doing. The sensory-seeking child is often attempting to fulfill a "sensory quota," so to speak, which means that if you are able to meet the child's quota, you should see a marked decrease in impulsive behaviors. Here are a few strategies to satisfy a child's need for sensory input:

- Hard running in the playground or running up stairs before class and at lunch time
- Daily PE class
- Moving desks around the classroom when appropriate
- Heavy-lifting tasks
- Putting on a weighted backpack for up to twenty minutes before a stressful event
- Therapeutic listening

Q. If we are adopting internationally, should we be concerned about SPD?

A. The sensory issues with adopted children are varied because there are so many factors involved, including nervous system maturation at birth, prenatal care (which many adoptive parents have no information about), and early experiences. You must also consider whether or not the child was in foster care or an orphanage. The conditions of the orphanage, including nutrition, outdoor time, and caregiver interaction, have an impact on your child's sensory processing. If you adopt internationally, you should be conscious of sensory processing issues.

Children from institutionalized backgrounds, such as orphanages or long-term hospital stays, have often experienced sensory deprivation and may have emotional or bonding issues. They have been deprived of the calming and nurturing sensory input that is crucial for a developing infant. The early input (proprioceptive, tactile, auditory, and vestibular) we receive as infants is what helps organize our nervous systems for more intense sensory input later in life. Neurochemicals are released by the brain that in turn releases hormones that have a calming or integrating impact on us; without those, we are more likely to feel stress. Children who have been institutionalized may have eating difficulties caused by oral sensitivities. Sensitivity to smell could result in an overactive gag reflex and lead to a disinterest or fear of eating.

Q. Are specific sensory issues more prevalent in children from certain countries?

A. The issues a child may have are more closely related to early life experiences than country of origin. However, there are generalized lifestyle differences and trends that may be a consideration for children from different countries. For instance, Russian women tend to consume more alcohol while pregnant, as evidenced by the rate of children born in that country with FASD, which is considerably higher than the world average. Research on primates has shown that even moderate alcohol consumption by the pregnant mother has an impact on sensory processing of the infant. In Central and South America, many of the babies are in foster care rather than in institutions, so there is more one-to-one attention, and they tend to carry the child everywhere. This is a positive as well as a negative—the infant gets lots of vestibular (balance and movement) types of activity plus more tactile and proprioceptive input, but less practice moving his own body against gravity, which is crucial for nervous system development.

Q. We just adopted our child from an orphanage in China. If she's sixteen months old and can't walk, should we be concerned that she has motor difficulties?

A. Not necessarily. Just remember that in the orphanage she probably did not have a reason to walk. It sounds odd but it's true. One of the key reasons a child begins to move is for cognitive exploration. In some orphanages, there may not be a reason to move to explore. Furthermore, caretakers may bring everything to the child—food, limited toys, and comfort. She does not need to move to seek things out. Therefore, when you bring her home, you may have to teach her how to want to move toward something. In some Central American countries, the child may not have had very many opportunities to walk because the foster family may not have put the child on the floor to explore. In this region of the world, parents tend to carry their children during much of their infancy.

Q. If my internationally adopted daughter has some sensory and motor issues, does that mean she has SPD?

A. Many times the behaviors you see in children who have been adopted from institutions can be referred to as "exposure delay." In orphanages, the light is usually dimmer, there is less auditory input, very few opportunities for movement are present, and there is little variety in diets. Children may not have been exposed to certain sensory experiences; thus, their nervous systems may perceive these new experiences as scary.

Q. Is there any link between children with reactive attachment disorder and SPD?

A. Before bonding becomes cognitive or something you think about as "I trust this person," bonding is all sensory. Think about what happens between a new infant and its primary caregivers. There is auditory input in the form of soft melodic words that are comforting, vestibular and proprioceptive input in the form of the deep-pressure and calming touch created by holding and rocking the infant, and controlled visual input from the faces of the caregivers continuously interacting with the new infant. These interactions all allow for a deep sense of trust to develop—the sensory input provided by the caregiver to the infant, the sensory experiences shared by both the infant and the caregiver, and finally the caregiver responding to the sensory needs of the infant. So when this is missing in those early months and years, the basis for trusting a person may not be there. Sensory integration therapy should be a large part of therapy geared toward children with reactive attachment disorder. Simply talking cannot make up for the missing sensory experiences!

Q. Is there anything I can do to help my adopted child "undo" her first year in the orphanage?

A. Yes, most children respond very well to comforting sensory input, as well as gradual introduction to new sensory experiences. You may have heard of the term "brain plasticity," which describes the nervous system/brain's ability to adapt and change to new information. This should be reassuring to adoptive parents. It is crucial to give your newly adopted child (no matter the age) a lot of the early sensory input that is paramount to bonding, such as deep and gentle touch, rocking, and lots of comforting auditory input, along with overexaggerated facial expressions.

If you have an older child, try having "baby time," where your child gets to be a baby for a certain amount of time, just so she can experience being a baby. You can also practice rituals that involve sensory input from parents, such as hair brushing, massaging arms, or rubbing feet. When you are exposing a child to what may be a new sensory input, remember to use deep pressure. For example, rub your child's shoulders before you push her on a swing or have her touch something she may be overly sensitive to.

Because movement is so crucial to our brain and body development, make it a priority for your child. Pay close attention to any sign of fear when your child's feet leave the ground. Many adopted children have gravitational insecurities due to a lack of early vestibular input in institutions. This issue should be addressed as soon as you become aware of it.

Chapter 16

THERAPEUTIC ACTIVITIES

- What are some vestibular activities I can do with my child?
- What are some proprioceptive activities I can do with my child?
- What are some tactile activities I can do with my child?
- What are some things I can do to strengthen my child's shoulders and hands?
- Are there activities that can help my child develop better praxis skills?
- What are some prewriting activities my child can do at home?
- What are some activities to help my child cross midline (the center of the body) and develop hand dominance?
- What are some activities my child can do at home that promote visual skills and visual motor skills?

Q. What are some vestibular activities I can do with my child?

A. Caution must be taken when engaging in activities that are designed to stimulate the vestibular system. Please refer to Chapter 6 for specific precautions. Here are some equipment-based activities to try:

- A "sit-n-spin" toy is a great way to introduce vestibular input to a younger child or a child that is very fearful of her feet being off the ground. With a sit-n-spin, children are still close to the ground and in most cases they control the amount of rotary input they receive.
- A balance board (www.abilitations.com) gives a child vestibular input while being close to the ground. A child can start out on his knees and then move to a standing position. As the child becomes more comfortable on the balance board, you can layer on other activities, such as playing catch or scanning the room to find an object. Also, try the Dizzy Disc Jr., an adjustable spinning and balancing ride toy.
- An exercise ball is probably the easiest to obtain and the most versatile tool you can use for vestibular and proprioceptive input. For very young children, you can place the child on the ball while holding her trunk while you move her from side to side. This helps develop core strength as well as develop "righting" reflexes. As a child gets older, you can have her sit on the ball while playing catch. It is also good to get kids on their bellies on the ball, reaching for items in front of them.
- Encourage activities on a trampoline (make sure to take safety precautions). This provides both proprioceptive and vestibular input.
- Swing equipment such as a hammock, flat swing, or Lycra swing (what OTs refer to as "suspended equipment") offers the most

powerful vestibular input you can give the nervous system. You can make a swing at home by using high-grade Lycra with loops or knots that attach it to a swivel.

- Have your child lie on his stomach on a scooter-board, which is simply a flat board with wheels, and have him hold on to a hula hoop as you pull him around. This activity also builds upper body strength.
- Encourage your child to swing; any kind of swing provides vestibular input. A tire swing is great because it goes in all directions.
- Get your child involved in activities that use pushing and pulling equipment, such as using a wheelbarrow, toy lawn-mowers, and so on.
- Get your child to practice walking with stilts; it gets his feet off the ground. Hippity hops and pogo sticks are another great way to get your kid's feet off the ground. This is a great reason to bring back toys from the era before computers and video games.
- Riding horses is a great way to promote healthy vestibular development.
- Bikes, trikes, and scooters help improve a child's sense of balance. These activities also promote both sides of the body working together in a coordinated manner.

Therapy equipment can be very costly, and there are alternatives that are less expensive. Here are some vestibular activities that require no equipment:

- More and more tummy time for your baby. This sets him up for experimenting with gravity and movement in the early months. It also helps strengthen the shoulders, neck, and arms, while providing much-needed proprioceptive input to the palmer surface of the hands.

- Cartwheels are appropriate for older children.
- Have your child roll down a grassy hill and, if desired, he can be wrapped in a large beach towel. (This is good for children age three and up.)
- Log rolls—have your child keep arms close to her side and roll on the floor.
- Pretzel—sit on the floor, cross your legs, and hold both feet. With your legs tucked, lean to the right until your elbow touches the floor. Roll onto your back, and continue rolling until you get to the point where your left elbow can push you up.
- Elephant—put your left ear on your shoulder and raise your left arm to look like a trunk. Using the pointer finger on the left hand, draw figure eights while your eyes focus on the tip of the finger doing the drawing.
- Rocking chair—sit on the floor, tuck your arms around your legs in front, and rock back and forth.

Have the whole family move their bodies to a rhythm/beat. Have everyone invent their own new dance moves that require the whole body to move in all directions!

Q. What are some proprioceptive activities I can do with my child?

A.
- Crashing into big soft objects (pillows, cushions)
- Resistance exercises (push-ups, pull-ups, carrying laundry, sit-ups)
- Playground activities, especially anything that involves climbing and pulling up

- Bounce on exercise ball
- Thera-band/tube exercises
- Animal imitations: bunny or kangaroo hop, frog jump, spider walk
- Boot camp exercises: obstacle course, army crawl
- Get your child involved with household chores, such as vacuuming, carrying groceries, raking leaves, and carrying laundry in the laundry basket.
- Encourage your older children (age four and up) to crawl around with something on their back, like a sack filled with rice or beans, or a pillow case filled with beanie babies.
- This one is easy! Give your child big bear hugs because these increase proprioceptive messages from the joints and tendons to the brain and help increase body awareness.
- Spandex body bags and whole-body squeezes can provide hours of entertainment (www.therapro.com and www.abilitations.com).
- Have your child carry objects of different weight.
- Encourage your child to open her own doors and yours, too!

Q. What are some tactile activities I can do with my child?

A.
- Play-Doh
- Draw pictures and letters in shaving cream, pudding, etc.
- Encourage sand or water play because it provides varying tactile experience.
- Make mud pies.
- Brushing protocol
- Hide paper clips in rice and find them.
- Find hidden object in Play-Doh, Thera-putty.

- Play a game where your child identifies different objects that you put in his hand while his eyes are shut, such as a penny or paperclip.
- Use fingers to draw letters on each other's backs and identify the letter.
- Brush skin with brushes of varying softness/stiffness, first self-brushing followed by partner brushing.
- Prepare food at home with varying degrees of messiness.

Q. What are some things I can do to strengthen my child's shoulders and hands?

A.
- Try push-ups against a wall to increase upper body strength.
- Hide coins in Thera-putty and have your child look for them.
- Give your child bubble wrap to pop.
- Encourage wheelbarrow walking—hold a young child around the hips or an older child by the knees or ankles and then make a game of seeing how far she can walk on her hands.
- Practice tunnel crawling.
- Cut Play-Doh with scissors.
- Use a plant sprayer to spray plants (indoors or outdoors) and also to spray snow. Mix food coloring with water so that the snow can be "painted."
- Pick up objects using large tweezers, tongs, or children's chopsticks—this can be adapted by picking up Cheerios, small cubes, small marshmallows, pennies, and so on, in counting games.
- Shake dice by cupping the hands together, forming an empty air space between the palms.
- Use small-sized screwdrivers like those found in an erector set.

- Lacing and sewing activities such as stringing beads, Cheerios, macaroni, and so on
- Use eye droppers to "pick up" colored water for color mixing or to make artistic designs on paper.
- Roll small balls out of tissue paper, then glue the balls onto construction paper to form pictures.
- Turn over cards, coins, checkers, or buttons, without bringing them to the edge of the table.
- Make pictures using stickers or self-sticking paper reinforcements.
- Play games with the "puppet fingers" (the thumb, index, and middle fingers).
- Take a tennis ball and make him into a smiling face with a slit cut for his mouth, have your child hold the tennis ball with one hand and squeeze to keep his mouth open while he feeds the smiling tennis ball with the other hand.

Pocket Full of Therapy (www.pfot.com) has lots of great fine motor toys.

Q. Are there activities that can help my child develop better praxis skills?

A. Yes, there are activities that help develop and refine gross motor and fine motor praxis.

First, it is important to note that *all* activities that are new or done in novel ways or locations require praxis. For example, you can probably write your name with your eyes closed, but if you have to write it upside down, your brain has to rethink how your body will accomplish this. It is similar to having the ability to ride a bike on a flat surface and then taking up mountain biking—your brain and body now have to figure out a new plan.

Gross motor planning (praxis) activities

- Activities that require balance and provide intense propriocep-tive input help develop praxis.
- Obstacle courses encourage motor planning skills. They can be designed with the child's age in mind. Have your child partici-pate in designing the activities for the obstacle course.
- Walking figure eights or taped patterns on the floor while trying to catch a ball or hit a balloon requires divided attention.
- When jumping on a mini or regular trampoline, practice jumping and then freezing into specific poses, such as a cat or a table.
- Wheelbarrow walking is good for motor planning, strength-ening, and provides proprioceptive input. Hold a young child around the hips or an older child by the knees or ankles and then make a game of seeing how far she can walk on her hands.
- "Simon says" is a great game for motor planning: At first, let Simon demonstrate things as you say them so your child will get both verbal and physical directions. Then start just saying body movements, and let your child figure out how to move her body.
- Imitate animals: Do the elephant walk, the crab walk, the duck walk, the bunny hop, the horse trot, gallop, and so on.
- Do the crab walk, forward and backward.
- Practice throwing beanbags at stationary targets, then moving targets, and progress into moving while throwing at a stationary target and then moving while throwing at a moving target.
- Break down everyday activities such as dressing and meal time into several small steps.
- Play musical chairs using pillows instead of chairs.
- Play charades.

- Play songs that encourage movement with music ,such as Kidz Jamz Series from Happy Turtles (www.KidzJamz.com), "The Wiggly Scarecrow" by Coles Whalen (www.kidfoundation.org), "Jumpin' Jellybeans" and "Say G' Day" by Genevieve Jereb, OTR (www.sensorytools.net), and "28 Instant Songames" by Maboaublo and Barbara Sher.

Fine motor planning (praxis) activities

- Cooking activities are excellent for encouraging planning and sequencing and also provide opportunities for various fine motor skills.
- Provide blocks and more blocks.
- Provide any kind of play tools (let your child try to figure out how to use something before you jump in!).
- Form clay or Play-Doh into balls and letters of the alphabet.
- Drop coins into a piggy bank one at a time.
- Take a tennis ball and make it into a smiling face with a slit cut for the mouth. Have your child hold the tennis ball with one hand and squeeze to keep his mouth open while he "feeds" the smiling tennis ball with the other hand.
- Build Lego designs.
- String macaroni, buttons, and different sized beads.
- Move a marble across, up, and down a wall with the thumb, middle, and index finger.
- Have your child practice writing letters on a chalkboard with his eyes closed.
- Provide toy nuts and bolts that require wrist rotation and finger manipulation.
- Screw and unscrew tops of jars, which helps with wrist rotation and motor planning.

- Put the caps back on markers.
- Spin a pinwheel.
- Play potato head, which includes lots of fine motor planning.
- Dress and undress dolls.
- Play dress-up (fine and gross motor).

Q. What are some prewriting activities my child can do at home?

A.

- Attach a large piece of drawing paper to the wall. Have the child use a large marker and try the following exercises to develop visual motor skills:
  - Make an outline of one figure at a time. Have the child trace over your line from left to right, or from top to bottom. Trace each figure at least ten times. Then have the child draw the figure next to your model several times.
  - Play connect-the-dots. Again, make sure the child's strokes connect the dots from left to right, and from top to bottom.
  - Trace around stencils—the nondominant hand should hold the stencil flat and stable against the paper, while the dominant hand pushes the pencil firmly against the edge of the stencil. You may have to hold the stencil to keep it in place.
- Use Wikki Stix to create shapes and letters.
- Have your child write shapes and letters with her eyes closed.
- Use your finger to draw letters on your child's back and say, "guess what letter or shape that was?"
- Use a chalkboard instead of a white board when your child is first learning to write because it provides more proprioceptive input and increases motor memory for letter formation.
- Activities done on a vertical surface increase shoulder strength as well as promote good wrist positioning for writing.

- Paint at an easel.
- Have your child practice drawing shapes or letters in rice or shaving cream.
- Use cookie dough to form letters or shapes and then bake and enjoy!
- Use large chalk to draw very large letters on the sidewalk and then make a game of walking the letters.
- Use a spray bottle to make letters or shapes on the sidewalk.
- Turn the Magna Doodle upside down so that the erasing lever is on the top. Experiment with making vertical, horizontal, and parallel lines.

Q. What are some activities to help my child cross midline (the center of the body) and develop hand dominance?

A.

- Encourage your child to reach across the body for materials with each hand. You may need to engage the other hand in an activity to prevent switching hands at midline.
- Present materials at midline to encourage the natural development of hand dominance.
- Start making the child aware of the left and right sides of his body through spontaneous comments such as, "kick the ball with your right leg."
- Play imitation posture games like "Simon says" with across-the-body movements.
- When painting at easel, encourage the child to paint a continuous line across the entire paper, and also from diagonal to diagonal.
- Do Brain Gym activities, such as cross crawl, having your child touch hand or elbow to the opposite knee.
- Draw circles with both hands on opposite sides of the paper.

- Follow a lazy-eight pattern on a chalkboard, with arms together or drawing over it with a piece of chalk.
- Play "hit the balloon" with a medium-sized balloon and switching hands; have a child wear a band on the hand she is supposed to use and then hit the balloon to each side of the body while encouraging her to keep her body straight forward. Try this while she is sitting on a therapy ball!

Q. What are some activities my child can do at home that promote visual skills and visual motor skills?

A.

Visual skills

- Use a flashlight against the ceiling. Have the child lie on his back or tummy and visually follow the moving light from left to right, top to bottom, and diagonally.
- Find hidden pictures in books such as *Where's Waldo?*
- Catching balls while walking or running or swinging is a great way to challenge the vestibular/visual team
- Blowing cotton balls across a table with a straw
- Blowing bubbles and trying to catch them on the end of the wand (yes it does help your eye muscles!)
- Complete maze activities.
- Play "I spy."
- Put different stickers on a ball and have your child yell out the color or letter before it gets to him.
- Practice watching toy cars go down a track without moving the head, only the eyes.
- Take hikes. Look to the horizon and then watch the ants marching in the dirt below!

Eye-hand coordination

- Play table tennis.
- Throw bean bags/koosh balls into a hula hoop placed flat on the floor. Gradually increase the distance of the hoop.
- Play throw and catch with a ball. Start with a large ball and work toward a smaller ball. (Koosh balls are easier to catch than a tennis ball.)
- Practice hitting plastic bowling pins with a ball.
- Play "hit the balloon" with a paddle.

Chapter 17

RESOURCES

■ What are some additional books and resources about Sensory Processing Disorder and the other related conditions?

■ What are the best websites with information related to sensory processing disorder?

■ Where can I find more information on the programs mentioned in this book, as well as other programs?

■ What books are recommended to learn about attachment issues?

■ How can I get in touch with other parents who have children with SPD?

■ Can you recommend some books on autism?

■ Where can I purchase equipment to help my child who has SPD?

■ What are some good websites for more information on autism?

Q. What are some additional books and resources about Sensory Processing Disorder and the other related conditions?

A.

- *Sensational Kids,* Lucy Jane Miller
- *Out of Sync Child,* Carol Kranowitz
- *The Out of Sync Child Has Fun: Activities for Kids with Sensory Integration Dysfunction,* Carol Kranowitz
- *Raising a Sensory Smart Child,* Lindsey Biel and Nancy Penske
- *An Introduction to "How Does Your Engine Run?"/The Alert Program for Self-Regulation,* Mary Sue Williams and Sherry Shellenberger
- *The Sensory Sensitive Child,* Karen Smith and Karen Gouze
- *The Everything Parent's Guide to Sensory Integration Disorder,* Terri Maurok
- *Answers to Questions Teachers Ask about Sensory Integration,* Carol Kranowitz, Stacy Szklut, et al.
- *Social Story Book—Illustrated,* Carol Gray
- *Writing Social Stories Video,* Carol Gray

Q. What are the best websites with information related to sensory processing disorder?

A.

- www.spdnetwork.org—provides a wealth of information, resources, and contacts completely dedicated to SPD.
- www.babystepstherapy.com
- www.sensoryint.com—another wealthy source of information; also, Sensory Integration International has a very useful database for finding clinics and therapists nationwide that specialize in sensory issues.
- www.otawatertown.com

- www.kid-power.org
www.sensory-processing-disorder.com
www.henryot.com

Q. Where can I find more information on the programs mentioned in this book, as well as other programs?

A.

- How Does Your Engine Run?—www.alertprogram.com
- Brain Gym—www.braingym.com
- Therapeutic Listening—www.vitallinks.net
- The Interactive Metronome—www.interactivemetronome. com
- Floor Time—www.floortime.com
- Eyes on Track—www.eyesontrack.com
- Handwriting Without Tears—www.hwtears.com; www. VisualLearnersAlphabet.com
- Core Concepts in Action—www.vitallinks.net
- Astronaut Training—www.vitallinks.net
- SCERTS (Social Communication, Emotional Regulation, and Transactional Support)—www.scerts.com

Q. What books are recommended to learn about attachment issues?

A.

- *When Love Is Not Enough: A Guide to Parenting Children with RAD (Reactive Attachment Disorder)*, by Nancy L. Thomas
- *Facilitating Developmental Attachment: The Road to Emotional Recovery and Behavioral Change in Foster and Adopted Children*, by Daniel A. Hughes

- *Attaching in Adoption: Practical Tools for Today's Parents,* by Deborah D. Gray
- *Building the Bonds of Attachment: Awakening Love in Deeply Troubled Children,* by Daniel A. Hughes

Q. How can I get in touch with other parents who have children with SPD?

A. The SPD network has a strong parent connection, with more than thirty-five parent support groups throughout the country. If there is not one in your area, you can ask your child's occupational therapist if you can post a sign in the clinic asking parents if they would like to get together for an "SPD over Coffee" support group. This will give you an idea of how many people are interested and then you can branch into postings in other clinics in your area. It is highly likely that other parents would welcome a support group of parents who are facing the same issues.

Q. Can you recommend some books on autism?

A.

- *The Autism Sourcebook: Everything You Need to Know About Diagnosis, Treatment, Coping, and Healing* by Karen Siff Exkorn
- *Helping Children with Autism Learn: Treatment Approaches for Parents and Professionals* by Bryna Siegel
- *Overcoming Autism* by Lynn Kern Koegel and Claire Lazebnik
- *The Autism Answer Book* by William Stillman
- *Let Me Hear Your Voice* by Catherine Maurice
- *Children with Autism: A Parent's Guide* by M. Powers
- *Teaching Children With Autism Strategies to Enhance Communication and Socialization* by K. Quill

Q. Where can I purchase equipment to help my child who has SPD?

A.

www.abilitations.com
www.specialkidszone.com
www.equipmentshop.com
www.integrationscatalog.com
www.jump-in-products.com
www.new-vis.com
www.pfot.com
www.pdppro.com
www.sensoryresources.com
www.southpawenterprises.com
www.sprintaquatics.com
www.talktoolstm.com
www.theraproducts.com
www.weightedwearables.com
www.vitallinks.com
www.sensorytools.net
www.sensorycomfort.com
www.superduper.com

Q. What are some good websites for more information on autism?

A.

- Autism Research Institute—www.autism.com/ari/
- Autism Society of American—www.autism-society.org
- Cure Autism Now Foundation—www.cureautismnow.org
- Families for Early Autism Treatment—www.feat.org
- Organizations run by autistic people—www.autistic.org

- O.A.S.I.S. (Online Asperger Syndrome Information Support)—www.udel.edu/bkirby/asperger
- Association for Positive Behavioral Support (APBS)—www.APBS.org
- Association for Behavior Analysis (ABA) www.abainternational.org

Appendix A

Sensory Diet

Date ———————————— Name ————————————

School ———————————— Age ————————————

Time	Key Events in the Day	Support Sensory Diet Activities	Comment / Sign Off

————————————————————

OT Signature

————————————————————

Teacher Signature

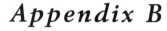

Appendix B

BEHAVIOR FLOWCHART

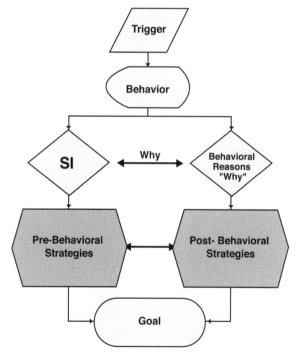

Delaney & Delaney 2006

Bibliography

Chapter 1

Ahn, R., L. Miller, S. Milberger, and D. McIntosh. (2004). Prevalence of parents' perceptions of sensory processing disorders among kindergarten children. *Am J Occup Ther* 58(3), 287–302.

Ayres, Jean. (1979). *Sensory Integration and the Child.* (Los Angeles: Western Psychological Services).

Foster, S., and T. Verny. *The development of sensory systems during the prenatal period. Journal of Prenatal and Perinatal Psychology and Health.*

Kranowitz, Carol Stock, and Lucy Jane Miller. (2006). *The Out-of-Sync Child: Recognizing and Coping with Sensory Processing Disorder.* New York: Perigee.

May-Benson, T.Sc.D. A theoretical model of ideation in praxis.(2007). In S. Roley, E. Banche, & R. Schaaf (Eds.), *Understanding the nature of sensory integration with diverse populations.* San Antonio: Therapy Skill Builders.

Miller, Lucy Jane. (2006). *Sensational Kids—Hope and Help for Children with Sensory Processing Disorder (SPD).* New York: Perigee.

Chapter 2

Biel, Lindsey, and Nancy Peske. (2005). *Raising a Sensory Smart Child*. New York: Penguin Group.

Frick, Shelia, and C. Hacker. (2000).*Listening with the Whole Body*. Madison: Vital Links.

Howard, Pierce Jo. (2006). *The Owner's Manual for the Brain, Everyday Applications from Mind-Brain Research*. Austin: Bard Press.

Lawton-Shirley, N., and P. Oetter. (2005). Sensory integration & beyond: Power tools for Treating children. Seminar: San Francisco.

Liddle, Tara, and Laura Yorke. (2004). *Why Motor Skills Matter.* San Francisco: Contemporary Books.

Murray-Slutsky, Carolyn, and B. Paris. (2005). *Is It Sensory or Is It Behavior?* San Antonio: PsychCorp.

Ratey, John. (2001). *A User's Guide to the Brain*. New York: Vintage Books.

Sunderland, Margot. (2006). *The Science of Parenting.* New York: DK Publishing.

Wynsberghe, D., and C. Noback. (1995). *Human anatomy & physiology* (3rd ed.). New York: McGraw-Hill.

Chapter 3

Hillier, Carl, and Mary Kawar. Eyesight to insight; Seminar: San Francisco.

Mailloux, Z. (1996) Play and the sensory integrative approach. In L. D. Parham & L. Fazio (Eds.), *Play in occupational therapy for children*. Boston: Mosby.

Remick, K. (2000). *Eyes on Track*. Folsom, CA: JF Publishing.

Richard, G. (2001). *The Source for Processing Disorders*. East Moline, IL: LinguiSystems.

Chapter 4

Apel, K., and J. Masterson. (2001). *Beyond Baby Talk*. New York: Three Rivers Press.

Oetter, Patricia, Eileen Richter, and Sheila Frick. (1995). *M.O.R.E: Integrating the Mouth with Sensory and Postural Functions* (2nd ed.). Stillwater, MN: PDP Press.

Schwentker, E. (2007, October). Toe walking. Available online at www.emedicine.com/orthoped/topic451.htm.

Chapter 5

Blanche, Erna, Tina Botticelli, and Mary Hallway. (1998). *Combining Neuro-Developmental Treatment and Sensory Integration Principles: An Approach to Pediatric Therapy*. San Antonio Therapy Skill Builders.

Bruininks, Robert. (1978) *Bruininks-Oseretsky Test of Motor Proficiency: Examiner's manual*. Circle Pines, MN: American Guidance Services.

Bundy, Anita, Shelly Lane, Anne Fischer, and Elizabeth Murray. (2002). *Sensory Integration Theory and Practice*. Philadelphia: Davis Company.

Case-Smith, Jane. (1998). *Pediatric Occupational Therapy and Early Intervention*. Philadephia: Butterworth-Heinemann.

Case-Smith, Jane. (2004). *Occupational therapy for children*. Boston: Mosby.

Chapter 6

Ayres, Jean. (1989). *Sensory Integration and Praxis Test Manual*. Los Angeles: Western Psychological Services.

Bundy, Anita, Shelly Lane, Anne Fischer, and Elizabeth Murray. (2002). *Sensory Integration Theory and Practice*. Philadelphia: Davis Company.

Dennison, P., and G. Dennison. (1994). *Brain Gym® teachers edition*. Ventura, CA: Edu-Kinsthetics.

Frick, S., and M. Kawar. (2004). *Core concepts in action*. Madison, WI: Vital Links.

Chapter 8

Baldi, H., and D. Detmers. (2003). *Embracing play: Teaching your child with autism* [video cassette]. Woodbine House.

Biel, Lindsey, and Nancy Peske. (2005). *Raising a Sensory Smart Child*. New York: Penguin Group.

Chapter 9

Bundy, Anita, Shelly Lane, Anne Fischer, and Elizabeth Murray. (2002). *Sensory Integration: Theory and Practice*. Philadelphia: Davis Company.

Ernsperger, Lori, Tania Stegen-Hanson, and Temple Grandin. (2004). *Just Take a Bite*. Arlington, TX: Future Horizons.

Individualized education program (IEP). Available online at www.ed.gov/parents/needs/speced/iepguide/index.html.

Rehabilitation Act of 1973, Public Law No. 93–112, 87 Stat. 394 (Sept. 26, 1973), codified at 29 U.S.C. § 701.

United States Congress, House Committee on Education and the Workforce. Subcommittee on Education Reform. (2003). *IDEA: Focusing on improving results for children with disabilities*. Washington, D.C. : U.S. G.P.O

Chapter 10

Heller, Sharon. (2002). *Too Loud, Too Bright, Too Fast, Too Tight: What to Do If You Are Sensory Defensive in an Overstimulating World*. New York: Harper Collins.

LeDoux, Joseph. (1996). *The Emotional Brain: The Mysterious Underpinnings of Emotional Life*. New York: Touchstone Books.

Chapter 11

Ahn, R., L. Miller, S. Milberger, and D. McIntosh. (2004). Prevalence of parents' perceptions of sensory processing disorders among kindergarten children. *Am J Occup Ther, 58*(3), 287–302.

Baker, Jed. (2003). *Social Training Skills.* Shawnee Mission, KS: Autism Asperger Publishing Company.

Bondy, Andy. (2002). *The Pyramid Approach to Education.* Newark, DE: Pyramid Education Products.

Dunn, W., J. Saiter, and L. Rinner. (2002). Asperger syndrome and sensory processing: A conceptual model and guidance for intervention planning. *Focus on Autism and Other Developmental Disabilities, 17*(3), 172–185.

Exkorn, Karen Siff. (2002). *The Autism Sourcebook.* New York: Regan Books.

Koegel, Lynn Kern, and Claire Lazebnik. (2004). *Overcoming autism.* New York: Penguin Books.

Miller, L. J., S. Schoen, J. Coll, B. Brett-Green, and M. Reale. (2005, February). *Final report: Quantitative psychophysiologic evaluation of sensory processing in children with autistic spectrum disorders.* Los Angeles, CA: Cure Autism Now.

Provost, B., B. Lopez, and S. Heimerl. (2006). A comparison of motor delays in young children: Autism spectrum disorder, developmental delay, and developmental concerns. *J Autism Dev Disord.*, Volume 37, Number 2, February 2007 , pp. 321–328(8).

Schetter, P. (2007). Best practice strategies and interventions for autism spectrum disorders. Course delivered at UC Davis, 2007.

Schneider, M. L., C. F. Moore, L. L. Gajewski, J. A. Larson, A. D. Roberts, A. K. Converse, and O. T. DeJesus. (in press). Sensory processing disorder in a primate model: Evidence from a longitudinal study of prenatal alcohol and prenatal stress effects. *Child Development.*

Siegel, Bryna. (2003). *Helping Children with Autism Learn.* New York: Oxford University Press.

William, Mary Sue, and Sherry Shellenberger. (1996). *How Does Your Engine Run?* Albuquerque: TherapyWorks Inc.

Chapter 12

Als, H., Gilkerson, L. Gilkerson, F. H. Duffy, G. B. McAnulty, D. M. Buehler, K. VandenBerg, N. Sweet, E. Sell, R. B. Parad, S. A. Ringer, S. C. Butler, J. G. Blickman, and K. J. Jones. A three-center randomized controlled trial of individualized developmental care for very low-birth-weight preterm infants: Medical, neurodevelopmental, parent and care giving effects. J Dev Behav Pediatr, 2003;24:399–408.

Index

About the Author

Tara Delaney, M.S., OTR/L, is a pediatric occupational therapist and founder of BabySteps, a pediatric therapy and educational services company (www.babystepstherapy.com). She conducts seminars internationally on sensory processing issues through the Making Sense-ory™ series. Tara is a graduate of the University of Texas Health Sciences Center and the University of Wisconsin-Madison.